Dysphagia in
Neuromuscular Diseases

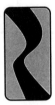

Clinical Dysphagia Series

John C. Rosenbek and Harrison N. Jones
Series Editors

Dysphagia Following Stroke by Stephanie K. Daniels and Maggie-Lee Huckabee
Dysphagia in Movement Disorders by John C. Rosenbek and Harrison N. Jones
Dysphagia Post Trauma by Elizabeth C. Ward and Angela T. Morgan
Dysphagia in Rare Conditions by Harrison N. Jones and John C. Rosenbek
Dysphagia in Neuromuscular Diseases by Robert M. Miller and Deanna Britton

Dysphagia in Neuromuscular Diseases

A Volume in the Clinical Dysphagia Series

Robert M. Miller
Deanna Britton

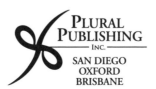

PLURAL
PUBLISHING
INC.
SAN DIEGO
OXFORD
BRISBANE

MW

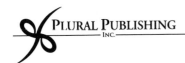

5521 Ruffin Road
San Diego, CA 92123

e-mail: info@pluralpublishing.com
Web site: http://www.pluralpublishing.com

49 Bath Street
Abingdon, Oxfordshire OX14 1EA
United Kingdom

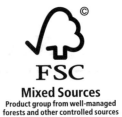

FSC
Mixed Sources
Product group from well-managed
forests and other controlled sources

Cert no. SW-COC-002283
www.fsc.org
© 1996 Forest Stewardship Council

Library of Congress Cataloging-in-Publication Data:

Miller, Robert M. (Robert Michael), 1946- author.
  Dysphagia in neuromuscular diseases / Robert M. Miller and Deanna Britton.
      p. ; cm. – (Clinical dysphagia series)
  Includes bibliographical references and index.
  ISBN-13: 978-1-59756-369-7 (alk. paper)
  ISBN-10: 1-59756-369-2 (alk. paper)
  1. Deglutition disorders–Diagnosis. 2. Deglutition disorders–Treatment. 3. Neuro-
muscular diseases–Complications. I. Britton, Deanna, 1962- author II. Title. III. Series:
Clinical dysphagia series.
  [DNLM: 1. Deglutition Disorders–diagnosis. 2. Deglutition Disorders–etiology.
  3. Deglutition Disorders–therapy. 4. Neuromuscular Diseases–complications. WI 250]
  RC815.2.M55 2011
  616.3'23–dc22

                                                                    2010054523

11/7/11

Contents

Foreword

Dysphagia in Neuromuscular Diseases by Robert Miller and Deanna Britton is a welcome addition to the four other books in the Clinical Dysphagia Series edited by J. C. Rosenbek and H. N. Jones. The books in this series are meant to be immediately clinically relevant: the relevance to reside in a combination of the best available data interpreted and supplemented by the best clinical experience and acumen. Complex, conceptually sound information was to be clearly summarized, and the art and science of swallowing management were to be highlighted. Authors were asked to write for busy clinicians with limited time for scholarship but with unlimited need to know and practice the best. *Dysphagia in Neuromuscular Diseases* succeeds on all counts.

The authors, in an excellent chapter on the clinical examination, applaud the "precious talent" of any practitioner capable of listening to the answers to the right questions and following up those answers with skilled evaluation and thoughtful interpretation. Clearly, these authors have that precious talent. As but one example, their chapter on the clinical examination could be used by even the most experienced clinicians as a gauge of their own clinical sophistication. New clinicians could launch their practices using the chapter's information as a guide. Indeed, all the chapters could serve these purposes, although Miller and Britton would probably be embarrassed by the suggestion. Each of their chapters contains reminders about the paucity of swallowing data in the neuromuscular disorders and, therefore, the need for clinical ingenuity. Their own ingenuity appears on every page.

These authors have another precious talent—they can write. This book is a pleasure to read. It is a hot air balloon ride sweeping the reader past the familiar—the videofluoroscopic swallowing examination and multiple sclerosis, and the less familiar—primary lateral sclerosis, polymositis, and the exotic-chronic inflammatory demyelinating polyneuropathy. Seeing these conditions from the authors' points of view will leave readers even more familiar with the procedures and conditions they know and ready to explore the ones they do not. Each chapter has clear landmarks: what could otherwise be impenetrable such as medical terminology is clarified, what could otherwise be a jumble such as the 30 or so types of muscle diseases is made orderly.

These authors are also courageous. They take measured and nondogmatic stands on many of the issues in modern dysphagia. For example, they remind us that the much maligned clinical swallowing examination is more likely to inform the clinician about the underlying pathophysiology of an individual patient's dysphagia than is the videofluoroscopic or endoscopic swallowing examination. On the other hand, the videofluoroscopic swallowing examination will provide unique information on structure and movement otherwise unavailable to even the most experienced clinician. As but one more example, they turn conflicting data about the appropriateness of treatment for conditions such as ALS into a structure of responsible clinical guidelines.

Clinicians have always shopped carefully for books, in part because book budgets are limited and because disappointment, especially with books advertised as clinical, is so frequent. This book will be money well spent. I predict the pages will get dog eared, the spine will get broken, the Table of Contents will get smudged, and owners constantly will be quizzing nonowners about the book's whereabouts.

John C. Rosenbek
Harrison N. Jones

Preface

The Yorkshire Dales of northern England, although pastoral, enchanting, and startlingly beautiful, can become a lonely place when you are stranded on a hillock, battered by wind and soaked by rain. You gaze out upon a stretch of boggy heather and thistle-covered moor; bleating sheep dot distant pastures; but no path is visible. At the trailhead, you were confident that the public footpath was clearly marked and pointed you toward your objective. But once out on the trail, markers were scarce and then nonexistent; you have lost your way. Standing ankle deep in the muck with no recognizable path forward or back, the dampness and chill contribute to your disorientation and bewilderment. Experience has proven, however, that with patience and a heavy dose of persistence you will discover a reliable path and find your way to your objective. Or, better yet, you may stumble upon the unexpected delight of a hospitable pub or the warmth of a local teahouse, and your discomfort will dissipate like the mist.

In agreeing to write this text, our assignment was clearly laid out. Our content editors, Drs. Rosenbek and Jones, could not have been more explicit: produce a "user-friendly" text that provides assistance to our fellow clinicians as they assess and treat individuals afflicted with neuromuscular disorders. They went so far as to provide us with an exemplar in their own work, *Dysphagia in Movement Disorders*. Dreaming of the fortune and worldwide acclaim that would inevitably flow from the completion of this work, we eagerly agreed to develop a volume that reflected our considerable clinical experience and our ability to synthesize vast amounts of research literature to provide guidance to our professional community. We were ready to pour out our wisdom vis à vis the clinical management of persons with neuromuscular diseases; we then would humbly bow to the applause.

Truthfully, we were neither that naïve nor that presumptuous. We did not begin this volume with the illusion that, in the process of our research and analysis, we would unravel some undiscovered mystery, once expressed, that would allow us to impart directions that would lead to the restoration of swallowing in persons afflicted with neuromuscular diseases. Like the majority of you who will use the information that follows, we are clinicians in heart and mind; we are realistic, grounded in our devotion to ethical practice, evidence, and continual learning.

With our assignment clear, we began the project with a reasonable degree of confidence. But, oh no, we must define neuromuscular disease! Bewilderment, indecision, and rapidly developing panic set in to create profound, overwhelming writer's block. Where to begin, and even more perplexing, where to end? The list of possible diseases/disorders was endless; many (truthfully most) were so rare that they were unfamiliar to us. There was no systematic classification system that had gained universal acceptance; indeed, there was no system that was truly comprehensible. We explored literature, discussed with colleagues, and meditated in an effort to realize some epiphany, some sense of enlightenment.

We wish that we could explain how we finally moved beyond the block and settled on what we conceived to be a comprehensible schema to review neuromuscular disorders. The fact is that you, the reader, will ultimately determine if we actually succeeded. Considering each disorder within its corresponding level of pathology did allow us to reflect on the physiologic relevance of treatment approaches. Furthermore, in compiling the information we present, we were forced to re-examine our own preconceived notions about the care we provide for individuals with various neuromuscular diseases.

Throughout the process of developing this volume, we constantly reminded ourselves that our ultimate goal was to make some contribution, although very indirectly, to the care of persons with neuromuscular disorders. We endeavored to communicate as clearly and relevantly as possible without making sacrifice to depth of knowledge. Our writing was guided by the same code that motivates us as clinicians—render care that is just, compassionate, and informed. It is to this latter notion that we have devoted our efforts; for it is our belief that knowing the disease is prerequisite to providing good care.

Michael Stipe, lead singer and songwriter for the rock group R.E.M., states, "Sometimes I'm confused by what I think is really obvious. But what I think is really obvious obviously isn't obvious." Returning to our imperfect analogy, we tried our best to provide you, our readers, with a path through the quagmire of neuromuscular disorders by providing obvious and conspicuous markers. We sincerely hope that, at the end of your exploration of this volume, you will find some sense of enlightenment. This may not in any way compare to the delight of discovering a friendly, rural Yorkshire pub or quaint village teahouse, but we trust that any knowledge gained ultimately will be applied to the benefit of your patients.

Robert M. Miller
Deanna Britton

Acknowledgments

RMM: My family—Nancy, Andrew, and Lindsey—whose love brings purpose, strength, and balance to my life. Special thanks to Andrew Miller, not just for his artistry, but for the patience and passion he brought to this collaboration.

DB: My husband, Tad, for his love and support.

We dedicate this volume to all those who have fought the battle with neuromuscular disease, especially James "Bud" Jones, and to those who read this work and provide the care.

1 Purpose and Scope

The purpose of this book is to offer guidance to clinicians in the evaluation and treatment of patients with oropharyngeal dysphagia resulting from degenerative neuromuscular diseases. Even a cursory review of the literature will demonstrate to practitioners that there are few data on oropharyngeal dysphagia as it is manifested in many of the neuromuscular diseases. With regard to providing interventions, clinicians most often are left with insubstantial guidance and a paucity of empirically supported treatment options. We aim to offer clinicians the best available evidence to support treatment decisions; however, lacking top-tier scientific research, we endeavor to provide as valid, consensus-supported, and clinician-observed guidance as possible. Ultimately, we are motivated to make a positive contribution to the lives of patients who live with neuromuscular diseases; it is to them that we dedicate this work.

To accomplish our purpose, we have operationally defined oropharyngeal dysphagia and discussed the critical interrelationships between the various stages of swallowing: oral, pharyngeal, and esophageal. In an effort to be thorough in our coverage we have proposed a methodology for the classification of neuromuscular diseases according to their level of pathology (Chapter 2).

Central to this text are chapters that provide foundational knowledge that is a prerequisite to understanding the pathologies of neuromuscular diseases. Clinicians who work with these patients and researchers who investigate diagnostic and treatment issues that pertain to these individuals need a clear understanding of the neurologic basis for swallowing, covered in Chapter 3. We have included three chapters (4, 5, and 6) that deal with various aspects of the assessment process that is applicable to patients with diseases in these categories. The clinical examination emphasizes the neurologic components of a focused head and neck inspection. Because muscular and neuromuscular diseases have a major impact on respiratory functions, we have included a chapter that provides the reader with a description of this physiologic system and describes tests that yield valuable data that is relevant to the treatment of these patients. Finally, there are caveats in the application of instrumental examination procedures that should be considered when assessing swallowing function in patients with neuromuscular disease.

Clinicians have a finite assortment of techniques that can be applied to patients with oral-pharyngeal dysphagia. For some interventions, there is strong evidence to support their application to achieve a defined physiologic effect. For example, when applied correctly, a prolonged swallow, or Mendelsohn maneuver, achieves longer airway closure along with other measurable changes in the swallow physiology. However, the choice of applying a given technique for a particular patient is not always clear and often there is not strong evidence to guide clinicians. In Chapter 7 we provide guidance based on principles of treatment as they apply to diseases and disorders found in the various levels of the neuromuscular system. Importantly, we endeavor to provide a framework from which clinicians can judge levels of evidence and effectively provide *evidence-based practice* to their patients.

It takes little effort to identify in the literature well over 1,000 different neuromuscular disorders when including variants in the presentation of syndromes and disparate etiologies. Any attempt to describe every disease, condition, disorder, or syndrome would be futile and foolish. How then can a book reasonably address this seeming potpourri of diseases that comprise the neuromuscular taxonomy? We have chosen to outline the various levels of the neuromuscular system, extending from the central nervous system (CNS) to the effector organ, or muscle, and develop chapters devoted to diseases that are representative of pathology at each level. For example, at the level of muscle pathology is a set of diseases defined as myopathies, and various forms of muscular dystrophy (MD) are representative. Stepping through the neuromuscular system, myasthenia gravis (MG) and Guillain-Barré syndrome (GBS) represent the levels of the neuromuscular junction and peripheral nerve respectively. Figure 1–1 illustrates the levels of pathology that extend from the upper

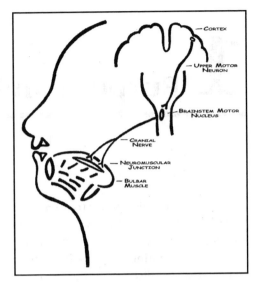

Figure 1–1. Levels of neuromuscular pathology. Levels of the neurologic systems include the axons of upper motor neurons extending from the cortex of the forebrain to synapse on a brainstem motor nucleus, and lower motor neurons originating in the pons and medulla with their axons bundled in the peripheral cranial nerve and synapsing at the neuromuscular junction of a bulbar muscle. Neuromuscular diseases are the result of pathology at one or more of these levels.

motor neurons originating in the cortex of the forebrain to the bulbar muscles that are utilized in swallowing.

For pathologies that are localized primarily within the CNS, the representative disease is not always a tidy fit. In the case of lower motor neurons, with cell bodies residing in the motor nuclei of the brainstem, degeneration is found in the presence of certain motor neuron diseases, amyotrophic lateral sclerosis (ALS) being the most prevalent. However, the pathology of ALS is not limited to the lower motor neurons; rather, by definition it also includes degeneration of upper motor neurons. Thus, although any text on neuromuscular diseases would be remiss in not addressing the details of ALS, this disease does not fit perfectly in any schema representing this classification of disease. Similarly, multiple sclerosis (MS), because of its prevalence, was chosen to represent upper motor neuron disease even though we recognize that the neural pathology is much more extensive and involves myelinated axons located throughout the CNS.

Regardless of the level of pathology, it is incumbent on every clinician to understand the nature of any disease or pathologic condition that they encounter. This volume endeavors to bring a clear perspective to a complex set of disorders, and in so doing, provide guidance for informed interventions to the treatment of dysphagia.

2 Definitions and Classification

This text deals with the impairment of dysphagia, or "disordered movement of the bolus from mouth to stomach due to abnormalities in the structures critical to swallowing or in their movements" (Rosenbek & Jones, 2009, p. 4). So as to provide readers with a perspective from which they can appreciate the impact of neuromuscular abnormalities on swallowing function, this chapter provides an operational definition for normal swallowing. Additionally, this chapter defines and classifies neuromuscular disorders from the standpoint of changes that occur in muscle tone and function as a result of pathology at each level of the nervous system. As the definitions and classifications for neuromuscular conditions and diseases are developed, the reader should keep in mind that there is no universally accepted classification system and that the various states of neuromuscular impairment rarely are pure. However, by understanding basic concepts we believe that clinicians will be able to relate impairments of swallowing function to particular neuromuscular conditions and, importantly, determine which treatment techniques make physiologic sense.

NORMAL SWALLOWING AND DYSPHAGIA: A BRIEF REVIEW

Normal swallowing involves the complex interactions of higher brain centers, sensory neurons, and motor systems of the central and peripheral nervous systems working to orchestrate the movement of a bolus from the mouth, through the esophagus, and into the stomach. To quote Rosenbek and Jones (2009, p. 3) in their companion text, *Dysphagia in Movement Disorders*, normal swallows are characteristically "safe, efficient, and satisfying."

It is traditional to divide normal swallowing into stages: oral preparatory, oral, pharyngeal, and esophageal. Each stage can be described in terms of its temporal characteristics, its place in the sequence of events, the relative degree of voluntary control that can be exerted, and by the movements observed in the process. But, it also should be recognized that there is a significant overlap and interrelationship between the stages. Although it is appropriate to think about the oral preparatory and oral stages as under voluntary control, they commonly are performed in an unconscious manner. The pharyngeal stage, beginning once a bolus has passed the faucal pillars and entered the pharyngeal cavity, is much more automatic and generally beyond our ability to modify once it begins. Often, the oral and pharyngeal stages overlap, although in other instances the two stages are distinctly separate, with the pharyngeal stage not beginning until the bolus is contained in the hypopharyngeal region. In either case, as the bolus passes through the pharyngeal cavity and toward the upper esophageal sphincter (UES), the muscular sequences transpire in a predictable, patterned manner. The UES is induced to relax by neural inhibition and it is mechanically pulled open by laryngeal elevation, a critical pharyngeal stage event. The patterned oral-pharyngeal stages of swallowing are coordinated with the respiratory cycle, providing a period of swallow apnea during which the airway is closed off and protected from the bolus flow. The esophageal stage then begins with a typically strong recontraction of the UES muscles and the initiation of a subsequent involuntary peristaltic wave traveling the length of the esophagus. In Chapter 3, Neural Basis for Swallowing and Dysphagia, the physiology of swallowing is described in more detail.

The critical aspects of this description of normal swallowing are: (1) the entire act of swallowing requires exquisite timing and coordination, which can be disrupted by alterations in the integrity of muscle fibers and neuromuscular status; (2) swallowing is typically coordinated with the respiratory cycle and supported by normal respiratory defenses like coughing and the mucocillary escalator; and (3) what occurs upstream in swallowing can and does affect function down-

stream, and vice versa. This latter issue is illustrated by imagining a swallow mechanism with impaired oral control and oral transport that allows an ill-prepared bolus to enter the pharynx, thus eliciting ineffective airway protection and pharyngeal transit. It also is significant that a problem at the level of the UES can be the result of more specific muscular impairments in either the pharynx or esophagus. And, finally, problems with esophageal peristalsis are frequently manifested by pharyngeal delays and inefficiencies in subsequent swallows (Jones, Ravich, Donner, Kramer, & Hendrix, 1985).

For our discussion, dysphagia is defined as an impairment in the movement of a bolus from the mouth, through the esophagus, and into the stomach due to alterations in the relevant structures and/or impairments in the higher brain centers, sensory neurons, and/or motor systems that influence and control swallowing. Such a disturbance commonly will interfere with swallowing safety, efficiency, and satisfaction. Dehydration, malnutrition, pulmonary aspiration, and loss of pleasure associated with eating are but a few of the consequences of dysphagia.

MUSCULAR AND NEUROMUSCULAR DISEASE AND IMPAIRMENTS

Throughout the text the term neuromuscular is used as an adjective to modify nouns such as disease, syndrome, condition, and tone. The term describes the relationship between neurons and muscles and implicit in this definition is the notion that this relationship is dependent on continuous feedback between the nervous system and muscular system.

Thus, a neuromuscular disease refers to a pathologic state in which there is disturbance in the interaction between neurons and muscle fibers. Herein lies a dilemma: Should we be inclusive and list all diseases that are manifested by a disturbance between neurons and muscles, a list that would easily exceed 100 diseases? Or, should we be exclusive and only include representative conditions in which, for example, the disturbance exists in either the muscle fibers alone (e.g., muscular dystrophy) or in the peripheral junction of nerve and muscle (e.g., myasthenia gravis)? We have chosen to reach our objective along two convergent paths: The first path allows us to explore representative diseases that occur at each level of the nervous system beginning with the peripheral muscles and ending with myelinated upper motor neurons of the central nervous system. We have devoted chapters to diseases in which a primary manifestation is a change in either the muscle fibers or muscle response to a neural impulse. The second path, integrated into each of the disorder chapters, approaches neuromuscular conditions from the perspective of the various pathologic conditions that develop at each level. Although this certainly is the "road less traveled," it motivates us to analyze impairments from the standpoint of the effector organ's status relative to such issues as muscle tone, reflex behavior, and muscle strength and endurance. Potential interventions, therefore, are considered from a physiologic perspective.

Muscle tone is defined as the amount of tension that exists in a muscle and this relates directly to the amount of resistance to movement that is present in the muscle. In normal conditions the central nervous system provides continuous, unconscious neural impulses to maintain a steady state of resistance. For skeletal muscles this means that there is sufficient resistance in both extensor and flexor muscles to maintain a normal posture. However, the muscles utilized for speech and swallowing functions differ in some important ways. Here the muscles must be able to perform actions that respond instantaneously to a neural impulse, whether it is an active contraction or inhibition. Especially in speech, but also with swallowing, structures like the tongue, lips, and vocal mechanism are capable of precise movements to preprogrammed target positions where they immediately release and adjust to another preprogrammed objective. Typically, the adjustment necessary to reach a subsequent posture or position begins even while the preceding motion is being completed. The normal steady-state tone in these oral-facial-pharyngeal-laryngeal muscles is, therefore, maintained to provide for these instantaneous responses to patterns of neural impulses.

In pathologic conditions the tone of muscles can be abnormally low, referred to as hypotonic, or high, hypertonic. For skeletal muscles abnormal tone is generally manifested by impaired posture. In hypotonic states, extensor muscles may fail to keep the body upright. In hypertonic states, there is an imbalance between the excitation and inhibition of agonist/antagonist, flexor/extensor muscles that interferes with smooth movement and normal posturing. For example, in the upper extremities the strong flexor muscles may be statically contracted, placing the arm in a constantly flexed posture. For muscles used to speak and swallow, hypotonia equates to a weakened state in which muscular structures either are incapable of reaching their programmed target positions or cannot maintain a posture for an adequate period of time. Hypertonia, on the other hand, may be manifested by slowness or the inability to rapidly adjust positions and postures. In either case, when the alteration in muscle tone is significant the functional consequence is abnormal speech and swallowing (dysarthria and oropharyngeal dysphagia).

The neuromuscular disorders described in this text are those for which abnormal muscle tone is often one of the major features. Specifically, we focus on those diseases and disorders that interfere with the actions required to swallow normally. As a consequence of the abnormalities in neuromuscular state, bulbar muscles are altered relative to their ability to initiate movements in a timely manner, to move smoothly and with precision, to move with adequate speed throughout a normal range of motion, and to exert adequate force while maintaining endurance. Impairments in one or more of these dimensions can and does interfere with the efficient and effective transfer of food and/or liquid from the mouth through the esophagus to the stomach. Many of the disorders discussed here are associated with a predictable direction of muscle tone change. For example, those conditions affecting lower motor neurons or any component of the motor unit (neuron, neuromuscular junction and muscle fiber) generally are associated with abnormally low muscle tone, hypotonicity or flaccidity. Myasthenia gravis, Guillain-Barré syndrome, and other neuropathies are disorders that lead to hypotonia. Conversely, upper motor neuron disorders like primary lateral sclerosis (PLS) and multiple sclerosis (MS) are associated with hypertonicity. Amyotrophic lateral sclerosis (ALS) by definition is a disease of both upper and lower motor neurons and leads to a combination of

hyper- and hypotonia, spasticity, and flaccidity. In this condition, the muscular tongue might have certain intrinsic and extrinsic muscles that are flaccid, with evidence of atrophic changes, whereas other muscles are spastic and incapable of moving with adequate speed and agility. Finally, a category of disorders labeled *cerebral palsy* (which is not specifically covered here) may present with either a single, characteristic tone (e.g., spastic, rigid, or flaccid CP), or an almost endless spectrum of muscle tone abnormalities (e.g., dystonic CP).

It is recognized that almost all diseases of the central nervous system will result in changes in neuromuscular status. Patients with Parkinson's disease (PD) or Huntington's disease (HD) will have muscle tone changes in the direction of increased resistance to passive stretch. PD, HD, and other diseases characterized by abnormal movements are addressed in the companion volume, *Dysphagia in Movement Disorders* (Rosenbek & Jones, 2009).

The preceding discussion describes the challenge inherent in defining neuromuscular disorders in such a way as to create reasonable boundaries. Our focus is on swallowing impairments that have as their basis a neuromuscular disorder. Impairments in muscle tone, strength, endurance, and to some extent coordination, are the physiologic consequence of these pathologies. We endeavor to discuss interventions that are appropriate for various neuromuscular states and approach specific disorders in an organized manner. Chapter titles designate a neurologic locus or level of pathology for disorders: muscular, neuromuscular junction, peripheral nerve, motor neurons, and myelinated axons of the central nervous system. For each level of the neuromuscular system, representative diseases and conditions are discussed, for example, muscular dystrophies at the level of muscle pathology. For each disorder we describe general aspects of the condition (e.g., signs/symptoms, pathology, and epidemiology), and concerns related to swallowing (e.g., swallowing pathology, assessment and treatment). We make every effort to present the best available evidence to support and guide practitioners, but are not timid about offering experienced-based guidance and judgments.

REFERENCES

Jones, B., Ravich, W. J., Donner, M. W., Kramer, S. S., & Hendrix, T. R. (1985). Pharyngo-esophageal interrelationships: Observations and working concepts. *Gastrointestinal Radiology, 10*, 225–233.

Rosenbek, J. C., & Jones, H. N. (2009). *Dysphagia in movement disorders.* San Diego, CA: Plural.

3 Neural Basis for Swallowing and Dysphagia

An understanding of normal swallowing and the manners with which it can be impaired by various neuromuscular disorders is critical for appropriate clinical intervention. In this chapter we briefly describe the anatomy and physiology of normal swallowing and then review the neural basis for swallowing with examples of how various neuromuscular conditions can affect the control and execution of swallowing. With recognition of these elements, clinicians will be in a better position to predict when and how swallowing will be affected and understand the rationale, or lack thereof, for applying various intervention techniques.

ANATOMY AND PHYSIOLOGY OF NORMAL SWALLOWING

The basic anatomy essential to oral-pharyngeal swallowing is illustrated in Figure 3-1. The following three conditions are typically met when swallowing: (1) The lips are sealed and the tongue tip elevated to prevent anterior leakage. An open-mouth swallow is possible, but difficult to perform. (2) The nasal passages are open to allow equalization of middle ear pressure through the eustachian tubes. Swallowing with the nares occluded is uncomfortable. (3) Oral mucosa is moistened by saliva. For most, a dry swallow without saliva cannot be performed.

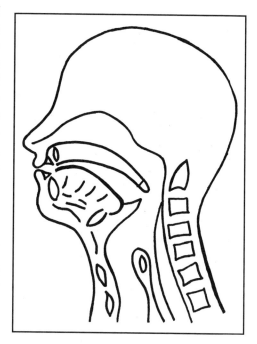

Figure 3–1. Anatomical structures for oral-pharyngeal swallowing. Oral-pharyngeal swallowing involves structures extending from the lips through the cervical esophagus and importantly includes the tongue, hard and soft palate, hyoid bone, epiglottis and entire laryngeal cavity, pharyngeal cavities from the nasopharynx through hypopharynx, and the muscular upper esophageal sphincter.

Figures 3–2, A through F, illustrate the stages of swallowing from oral through the early esophageal phase. It is critical that clinicians understand the sequence of events that occur as a bolus is actively evacuated from the oral cavity, transported through the pharynx, and into the esophagus. During this sequence note that the bolus is directed toward low-pressure zones, or expanding cavities, and away from high-pressure areas, those that are being sealed off or narrowed by contracting muscles. Consider, for example, nasopharyngeal regurgitation, a pathologic condition in which the velopharyngeal muscles have failed to adequately contract and create a high-pressure zone in the nasopharyngeal cavity. If the pressure in nasopharynx remains relatively low during the oral-pharyngeal stage of swallowing, the bolus most likely will be misdirected into this region. Other examples of bolus misdirection due to the failure to create a high-pressure zone are oral leakage from impaired lip seal and airway penetration due to inadequate laryngeal seal. Differential pressure zones are created throughout the oral and pharyngeal stages of swallowing by the rapid muscle contractions that are occurring to adjust the positions of anatomic structures. Thus, a bolus is evacuated out of the oral cavity, squeezed through the oro- and hypopharynx, and passed through the upper esophageal sphincter and away from the entrance to the airway. The sequence of active muscle contractions and subsequent inhibition found in

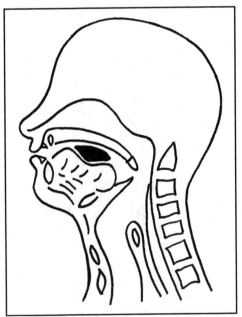

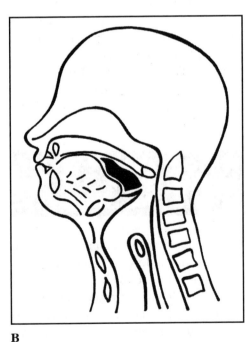

A   B

Figure 3–2. Oral-pharyngeal swallowing sequence. Once a bolus is prepared for swallowing, the bolus is **(A)** contained in the oral cavity by sealing the lips and elevating the tongue tip. The bolus is then **(B)** compressed between the tongue, hard palate and velum to move it toward the pharyngeal cavity and stimulate contraction of velar muscles to seal off the nasopharynx. *continues*

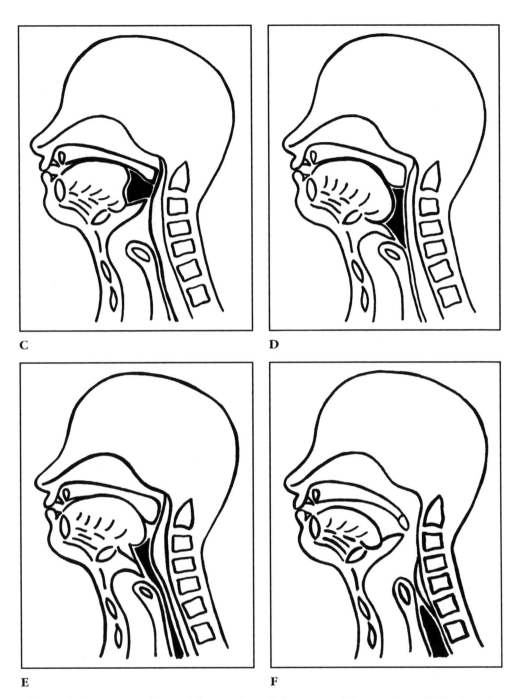

C

D

E

F

Figure 3–2. *continued* Forceful retraction of the tongue (**C**) propels the bolus into the pharyngeal cavity while pharyngeal contractions begin the process of stripping the bolus in the direction of the esophagus. Upon entering the pharyngeal cavity (**D**) muscles attached to the hyoid bone synchronously contract to move the larynx in an anterior-superior direction and "flip" the epiglottis over the entrance to the airway. At the height of the pharyngeal phase of swallowing (**E**), the combination of laryngeal elevation and inhibitory neural impulses allow the upper esophageal sphincter (UES) to relax its tonic contraction and to be mechanically pulled open. Once the bolus has been fully stripped through the UES (**F**), the muscles that comprise the sphincter contract strongly as esophageal peristalsis takes over to clear the bolus through the lower esophageal sphincter and into the stomach.

normal swallowing is not viewed as a series of distinct events, but rather appears as an orchestrated flow of movement in which the cavities involved are seamlessly reshaped and transformed by over 25 pairs of muscles to accommodate efficient bolus transport (Doty, 1968; Goyal & Cobb, 1981; Jean, 2001; Miller, 1982).

What occurs with the presence of neuromuscular disease can be thought of as a disruption in the timing and/or completeness of the movements necessary to bring about a smooth orchestration of muscle contractions. Although muscle weakness is the common denominator in almost all neuromuscular conditions, the effect on swallowing will differ depending on the nature of the condition. Some neuromuscular diseases, because of impairments in the inhibitory components of the central nervous system (CNS), will produce neuromuscular states that are analogous to stiffness, namely, the increased muscle tone of spasticity and rigidity (hypertonic muscles). Others will affect the biomechanics in the opposite direction primarily by impairing muscle force and endurance, these associated with flaccidity and low muscle tone (hypotonicity). Consider, for example, the effect that "stiffness" might have as a disrupting factor in the biomechanics of swallowing; conversely, "laxity" might be expected to have a completely different manifestation. For a patient with hypertonic muscles, we commonly observe ill-timed contractions and impaired control of boluses, particularly those that flow rapidly from the oral to pharyngeal cavities, for example, thin liquids. In hypotonic states, there is more likely to be a failure to achieve a complete muscle contraction that can result in observations such as the inability to maintain oral containment, velopharyngeal regurgitation,

airway penetration, and pharyngeal stasis. Identifying the nature of the neuromuscular state is therefore critical in the selection of appropriate interventions to ameliorate functional swallowing.

NEUROLOGY OF SWALLOWING

The neural control of swallowing involves many components, including: (1) a central nervous system (CNS) control unit located in the medulla, often referred to as the central pattern generator (CPG) for swallowing, or sometimes the swallowing center; (2) higher brain regions in the cerebral cortex that have the capability of signaling the CPG to voluntarily initiate a swallow; (3) motor control systems of the basal ganglia and cerebellum that serve to stabilize muscles and maintain normal muscle tone through a continuous flow and balance of excitatory and inhibitory impulses; (4) several peripheral cranial and spinal nerves that provide both the sensory (afferent) input to the CPG and motor (efferent) output from the CPG to execute the patterned muscle actions of swallowing; and (5) the muscles themselves which must be capable of responding to neural impulses by rapidly contracting and then relaxing to accomplish myriad configurations and adjustments required to efficiently and safely swallow. Presumably, a malfunction at any level could result in a neuromuscular impairment.

Swallowing Central Pattern Generator (CPG)

The CPG for swallowing is a set of bilateral nuclei located in the medulla oblongata of the brainstem that is primarily responsible for the involuntary elicitation of swallowing. The medullary swallowing centers largely have been defined on the basis of animal studies; however, a basic model that can be applied to humans has emerged from the available data. Structurally, the CPG is composed of at least two major nuclei within the medulla oblongata: the nucleus solitarius located dorsally and the nucleus ambiguus in the ventral region. These nuclei, along with adjacent medullary reticular nuclei, are represented on both sides of the medulla and they are interconnected (Doty, Richmond, & Storey, 1967; Lowell et al., 2008; Martin, 1989). The patterned muscle contractions and relaxations of the pharyngeal and esophageal stages of swallowing can be elicited from stimulation of nuclei on either side. The important clinical implication is that significant disruption of swallowing is associated with a unilateral medullary lesion on either side (Aviv, Mohr, Blitzer, Thomson, & Close, 1997).

In Figure 3–3, one set of paired medullary nuclei of the CPG are represented along with their afferent input and efferent output. Although these nuclei primarily facilitate involuntary (unconscious) swallows, they also participate in voluntary swallowing. Involuntary swallows are elicited when sensations arising from the properties of saliva, food, and/or liquid in the oral cavity (taste, touch, temperature, texture, pressure) are carried by cranial nerves V, VII, IX, and X and synapse on the dorsal nuclei. Voluntary, willful swallowing also can be elicited when higher cortical ("supramedullary" or "supranuclear") centers command the dorsal nuclei to respond. The dorsal nuclei, once stimulated from peripheral afferents and/or supranuclear centers,

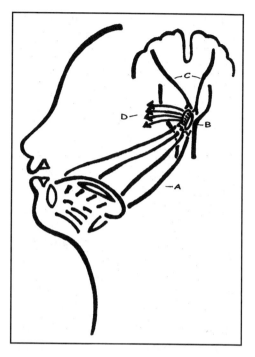

Figure 3–3. Central pattern generator for swallowing. The axons of peripheral afferent nerves (**A**) transmit neural impulses to paired nuclei of the medulla (**B**) that represent a *central pattern generator for swallowing* (CPG). The dorsal nucleus, or *nucleus solitarius*, can be activated by either the sensory input received via cranial nerves for automatic, unconscious swallowing, or from supramedullary impulses (**C**) originating in higher levels of the brain for voluntary swallowing. When activated, the dorsal nuclei signal the ventrally situated *nucleus ambiguus* which in turn distributes efferent impulses (**D**) to those motor fibers that must contract in a patterned manner to achieve safe and efficient swallowing.

activate the ventral nuclei of the CPG. In turn, the ventral nuclei distribute a complex, stereotyped pattern of motor impulses via cranial nerves V, VII, IX, X, XII, and cervical spinal nerves 1 through 3. The resulting movements involve the activation and inhibition of more than

25 pairs of muscles in the face, mouth, pharynx, larynx, and esophagus (Doty et al., 1967; Miller, 1982). It is important to note that the nuclei of the CPG for swallowing are physically located in the same sites as the CPG for respiration and cardiovascular regulation (Jean, 2001). Given that swallowing and respiration require exquisite coordination and use many of the same anatomic structures, the proximity of these systems is logical.

Cortical Swallowing Regions

The supranuclear (also supramedullary, supratentorial, or forebrain) areas capable of eliciting voluntary swallowing are primarily located in the frontal motor cortices of both hemispheres, anterior to the sensorimotor cortex (Jean & Car, 1979). Both hemispheres of the brain are capable of eliciting swallowing. In fact, discrete somatotopical representations of the swallowing musculature have been demonstrated using fMRI on the motor and premotor cortex of both hemispheres (Hamdy et al., 1996). Although the oral preparatory stage of swallowing is subject to voluntary control through the primary motor cortices, the primary motor areas do not appear to be involved during the patterned movements of the pharyngeal stage (Huckabee, Deecke, Cannito, Gould, & Mayr, 2003). In other words, unlike finger movements for example, there is no specific cortical motor point along the primary motor cortex from which one can elicit by stimulation the sequential contractions that occur during the pharyngeal stage of swallowing. Rather, evidence suggests that the patterned movements of pharyngeal swallowing are influenced by more disseminated indirect pathways connecting cortical motor planning areas to the brainstem motor neurons.

Additionally, there is support for interhemispheric asymmetry for swallowing. Important evidence suggests that lesions to either the left or right hemisphere result in distinctively different patterns of dysphagia. For example, left cortical stroke results in more oral stage impairment and initiation difficulties whereas right-sided vascular lesions are associated with inefficient swallowing and observations of pooling, airway penetration, and aspiration (Robbins & Leviue, 1988). Furthermore, there is evidence to suggest that during recovery from unilateral stroke the pharyngeal representation along the motor cortex in the intact hemisphere actually increases in size (Hamdy et al., 1996). Conversely, for the atypical patient with persistent dysphagia following unilateral stroke, no measurable increase in size for the representation of pharyngeal musculature is found (Hamdy, Rothwell, Aziz, & Thompson, 2000). The question of a dominant hemisphere for swallowing, although possible, remains open.

In addition to the frontal cortical areas just described, other regions of the supratentorial brain have been identified as being important to voluntary swallowing. Using imaging techniques, the insula, anterior cingulate gyrus, prefrontal cortex, anterolateral and posterior parietal cortex, and superiomedial temporal cortex, to list a few, are activated (Hamdy, Rothwell, Brooks, Bailey, Aziz, & Thompson, 1999; Kern, Jaradeh, Arndorfer, & Shaker, 2001). The sum of the available data suggests that swallowing is a multidimensional behavior involving many brain regions and pathologic conditions occurring at multiple cortical and subcortical sites result in changes in the swallowing mechanism.

Contributions from Motor Control Systems

It is well established that cortical areas maintain input to the medullary swallowing CPG and that this input is critical for voluntary initiation of swallowing. The cortical areas in turn are influenced by a near-constant flow of impulses from the basal ganglia and cerebellum, both of which serve to maintain stability and normalize tone in the muscular system, including the swallowing musculature. Taken together, the basal ganglia and cerebellum represent the motor control centers of the brain. Often pathologies in these motor control centers result in movement disorders and these conditions are thoroughly reviewed in the companion text, *Dysphagia in Movement Disorders* (Rosenbek & Jones, 2009).

Degenerative neurologic diseases that affect the function of nuclei of the basal ganglia can result in either hypokinetic abnormalities, such as rigidity and poverty of movement, or hyperkinetic abnormalities like chorea, dystonia, myoclonus, and dyskinesia. A classic example of hypokinetic impairment comes from Parkinson's disease (PD) in which cortical areas may not receive adequate excitation from the nuclei of the basal ganglia. The end result is that voluntary movements may not be efficiently initiated (e.g., impaired initiation of oral stage swallowing) and spontaneous movements may be diminished (loss of normal facial expression). On the other end of the continuum, Huntington's disease (HD) typically illustrates hyperkinetic features. Here there is insufficient inhibition of cortical motor areas originating from the basal ganglia resulting in unwanted, uncontrolled involuntary movements that disrupt the typical patterns of swallowing. For example, sudden inhalation might occur as the bolus traverses the pharynx and thus is redirected into the airway.

The contributions of the basal ganglia to the maintenance of normal muscle tone and movement are extremely complex, and the explanations for the pathologies of PD and HD provided here have been greatly simplified. The major nuclei of the basal ganglia are the striatum consisting of the caudate and putamen, and the external and internal globus pallidus. These nuclei have rich connections to other midbrain nuclei like the subthalamic and substantia nigra. Together, the basal ganglia and associated nuclei, communicate through circuit loops that transmit excitatory and inhibitory neural flow to cortical areas via the thalamus. Lesions affecting one or more of these circuits can potentially disrupt function in myriad ways. Whether by degeneration of nuclei or infarction (Kobayashi, Nakagawa, Sekizawa, Arai, & Sasaki, 1996; Logemann et al., 1993), swallowing patterns frequently are affected.

Brain mapping studies also have implicated components of the basal ganglia and cerebellum as active neurologic components in volitional swallowing (Suzuki, et al 2003). More specifically, the left hemisphere of the cerebellum has been identified as playing an important role in volitional swallowing (Hamdy et al., 1999; Harris et al., 2005). In their assessment of regional cerebral blood flow (rCBF) using PET imaging, Zald and Pardo (1999) measured activation of the cerebellum during swallowing and attributed this to a specific representation of the pharyngeal and esophageal regions. The authors point out that, although there are cases of dysphagia reported due to cerebellar lesions or atrophy, most of these involve widespread lesions that extend beyond the cerebellum itself. Recognizing the cerebellum's contribution to motor behavior in general, it is reasonable to conclude that the cerebellum assists in the timing, sequencing, and coordination of swallowing.

Peripheral Cranial and Spinal Nerves

Peripheral nerves are the pathways that connect sensory organs and musculature to the CNS. Peripheral cranial nerves are responsible for carrying afferent input to the CNS from the mucosa of the deglutitory tract. Sensory flow is critical for normal swallowing; generally, spontaneous swallows are generated by the sensations of touch, texture, pressure, and temperature. Similarly, all muscles involved in the act of swallowing are innervated by peripheral motor nerves either emanating from the brainstem as a cranial nerve (CN), or from the cervical spine as a spinal nerve (SN). Each peripheral nerve is referred to as *final common pathway* because it links a muscle to the CNS activation and control center. A complete lesion in a peripheral motor nerve will break this link and the corresponding muscle will be rendered flaccid and begin to atrophy. Flaccidity in one or more of the deglutitory muscles can result in a serious swallowing impairment. Table 3–1 summarizes the peripheral nerves and their contributions to swallowing.

Table 3–1. Peripheral Nerves Involved in Swallowing

Nerve	Sensory Function	Motor Function
CN V (trigeminal)	touch, pressure, and temperature from anterior 2/3 tongue, mucosa of the cheek, floor of mouth, hard palate, velum, and gums	muscles of mastication; controls jaw opening and closure
CN VII (facial)	taste from anterior 2/3 of the tongue	muscles of facial expression including the lips; sublingual and submaxillary salivary glands
CN IX (glossopharyngeal)	taste from the posterior tongue; touch, pressure, and temperature from mucosa of oropharynx, palatine tonsils and fauces, and posterior tongue	stylopharyngeus muscle; parotid gland
CN X (vagus)	senses mucosa of hypopharynx, epiglottis, and laryngeal cavity	pharynx and larynx; sympathetic fibers to the esophagus
CN XII (hypoglossal)		muscles of the tongue
SN 3–5 (cervical spinal nerves)		muscles of respiration

The CNs critical to carrying the sensations to generate swallowing are CNs V, VII, IX, and X. CN V carries the important afferent qualities of touch, pressure and temperature from the anterior two-thirds of the tongue and the mucosa of the cheek, floor of mouth, hard palate, velum, and gums. CN VII carries taste from the anterior two-thirds of the tongue. CN IX relays taste from the posterior tongue and other sensations (touch, pressure, and temperature) from the mucosa of the oropharynx, palatine tonsils and fauces, and the posterior tongue. CN X transmits sensations that are critical to both swallowing and airway protection; the senses derived from the mucosa of the hypopharynx, epiglottis and laryngeal cavity. Attention also should be paid to CN I, the olfactory nerve, because of the intimate relationship between taste and smell. These two sensory modalities combine to stimulate saliva production and secretion.

As has been noted, the motor system for swallowing involves over 25 pairs of muscles in the jaw, oral cavity, pharynx, and larynx, plus muscles of the esophagus and respiratory system (Doty, 1968; Goyal & Cobb, 1981; Jean, 2001; Miller, 1982). Each swallow requires a coordinated sequence of muscle activation and inhibition that involves several CNs (V, VII, IX, X, and XII) and SNs (3, 4, and 5). CN V innervates muscles of mastication and controls jaw opening and closure. CN VII, the facial nerve, supplies muscles of facial expression including the lips that are sealed during normal swallowing. CN VII is also important for its innervations of the sublingual and submaxillary salivary glands. The glossopharyngeal nerve, CN IX, and the vagus, CN X, usually are considered together in neurologic examinations, as they are difficult to separate out anatomically and functionally. CN IX innervates the stylopharyngeus muscle and carries efferent impulses to the parotid gland for salivary secretion. CN X innervates the somatic muscles of the pharynx and larynx and supplies sympathetic fibers to the esophagus. Although the peripheral CN XI, the spinal accessory nerve, innervates muscles not directly involved in swallowing, namely, the trapezius and sternocleidomastoid muscles, some fibers from the spinal accessory nucleus join the vagus to innervate portions of the pharynx and larynx. CN XII, the hypoglossal nerve, supplies the muscles of the tongue and thus is responsible for the lingual movements critical to swallowing. Finally, SNs emanating from cervical levels 3, 4, and 5 are essential in the innervation of muscles of respiration.

The Deglutitory Muscular System

Both striated somatic muscles (e.g., jaw, face, mouth, pharynx, larynx, and upper esophagus) and smooth visceral muscles (lower esophagus) are involved in swallowing. As described above, these muscles are innervated by peripheral nerves and controlled by the CNS. Pathology in the peripheral muscles results in serious impairment to swallowing, and although not strictly a neuromuscular impairment, in every operational and functional sense these muscle disorders mimic pathologies in the nervous system. For this reason, muscle pathologies, for example, myopathies are considered in the discussion of neuromuscular disorders.

Myopathy is a general term that describes either an acquired or inherited disorder and can result from endocrine, metabolic, infectious, or inflammatory conditions, particular drugs and gene mutations. Although symptoms of myopathy are most commonly experienced in the limb muscles, they certainly can be manifested in muscles essential for swallowing. The features found in certain forms of myopathy are weakness of facial and oral-pharyngeal muscles, decreased or absent reflexes, and stiffness or slowness in relaxing after a contraction. This latter symptom, found in some forms of muscular dystrophy, is referred to as myotonia. Fatigue, repeated contractions, and cold temperatures, all of which have implications for swallowing, can exacerbate it.

Neuromuscular Control and Execution of Swallowing

Most swallowing is involuntary and occurs automatically without awareness, at a frequency of a little over 1 swallow per minute on average for a typical adult. This form of swallowing can be considered to be a patterned motor response that is elicited at the brainstem level. These swallows are dependent on the integrity of the nuclei of the CPG for swallowing, the peripheral nerves, and the muscles themselves. Furthermore, the tone and contractile characteristics of the muscles are dependent on the balance of inhibitory and excitatory impulses that the brainstem nuclei constantly receive from higher brain centers. As illustrated in Figure 3–4, the brainstem receives impulses from both hemispheres of the brain and the preponderance of the input is inhibitory. When there is disruption of input from higher centers of the brain bilaterally, which would occur with bilateral hemispheric disease affecting motor con-

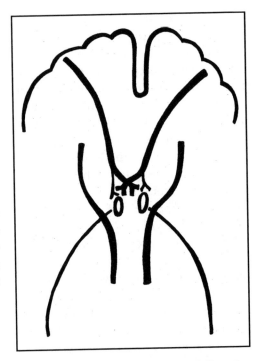

Figure 3–4. Bilateral corticobulbar input to brainstem motor nuclei. Brainstem motor nuclei receive both inhibitory and excitatory impulses from motor areas located in both cerebral hemispheres. Although the preponderance of motor control is contralateral and the degree of bilateral control varies across motor nuclei, all bulbar motor nuclei involved in swallowing receive some bilateral input.

trol systems, the lack of inhibition typically results in disorders characterized by hypertonicity (spasticity or rigidity). The likelihood of movement disorders and muscle instability is great when there is impairment in the motor control systems described above. Disruption at the level of the brainstem nuclei or lesions to peripheral nerves disconnects muscles from the CNS drive and the result is hypotonicity or flaccidity.

Voluntary swallows differ from involuntary with regard to the point of neurologic origin. In a voluntary swallow, drive originates primarily from the frontal lobes in either hemisphere sending initiatory impulses to the brainstem centers to trigger a swallow. Beyond this, the effectiveness of the swallow remains dependent on the integrity of the systems described above for an automatic swallow.

REFERENCES

Aviv, J. E., Mohr, J. P., Blitzer, A., Thomson, J. E., & Close, L. G. (1997). Restoration of laryngopharyngeal sensation by neural anastomosis. *Archives of Otolaryngology-Head and Neck Surgery*, *123*, 154-160.

Doty, R. W. (1968). Neural organization of deglutition. In C. F. Code & C.L. Prosser (Eds.), *Handbook of physiology, alimentary canal* (pp. 1861-1892). American Physiological Society, Washington, D.C.

Doty, R. W., Richmond, W. H., & Storey, A. T. (1967). Effect of medullary lesions on coordination of deglutition. *Experimental Neurology*, *17*, 91-106.

Goyal, R. J., & Cobb, G. W. (1981). Motility of the pharynx, esophagus and esophageal sphincters. In L. R. Johnson (Ed.), *Physiology of the gastrointestinal tract* (pp. 359-391). New York, NY: Raven Press.

Hamdy, S., Aziz, Q., Rothwell, J. C., Krishna D. Singh, K. D., Barlow, J., . . . Thompson, D. G. (1996). The cortical topography of human swallowing musculature in health and disease. *Nature Medicine*, *2*, 1217-1224.

Hamdy, S., Rothwell, J. C., Aziz, Q., & Thompson, D. G. (2000). Organization and reorganization of human swallowing motor cortex: Implications for recovery after stroke. *Clinical Science*, *99*, 151-157.

Hamdy, S., Rothwell, J. C., Brooks, D. J., Bailey, D., Aziz, Q., & Thompson, D. G. (1999). Identification of the cerebral loci processing human swallowing with $H_2^{15}O$ PET activation. *Journal of Neurophysiology*, *81*, 1917-1926.

Harris, M. L., Julyan, P., Kulkarni, B., Gow, D., Hobson, A., Hastings, D., . . . Hamdy, S. (2005). Mapping metabolic brain activation during human volitional swallowing: A positron emission tomography study using [^{18}F]fluorodeoxyglucose. *Journal of Cerebral Blood Flow and Metabolism*, *25*, 520-526.

Huckabee, M., Deecke, L., Cannito, M. P., Gould, H. J., & Mayr, W. (2003). Cortical control mechanisms in volitional swallowing: The Bereitschaftspotential. *Brain Topography*, *16*, 3-17.

Jean, A. (2001). Brain stem control of swallowing: Neuronal network and cellular mechanisms. *Physiological Review*, *81*, 929-969.

Jean, A., & Car, A. (1979). Inputs to the swallowing medullary neurons from the peripheral afferent fibers and the swallowing cortical area. *Brain Research*, *78*, 567-572.

Kern, M. K., Jaradeh, S., Arndorfer, R. C., & Shaker, R. (2001). Cerebral cortical representation of reflexive and volitional swallowing in humans. *American Journal of Physiology, Gastrointestinal and Liver Physiology*, *280*, G354-G360.

Kobayashi, H., Nakagawa, T., Sekizawa, K., Arai, H., & Sasaki, H. (1996). Levodopa and swallowing reflex. *Lancet*, *348*, 1320-1321.

Logemann, J. A., Shanahan, T., Rademaker, A. W., Kahrilas, P. J., Lazar, R., & Halper, A. (1993). Oropharyngeal swallowing after stroke in the left basal ganglion/internal capsule. *Dysphagia*, *8*, 230-234.

Lowell, S. Y., Poletto, C. J., Knorr-Chung, B. R., Reynolds, R. C., Simonyan, K., & Ludlow, C. L. (2008). Sensory stimulation activates both motor and sensory components of the swallowing system. *NeuroImage*, *42*, 285-295.

Martin, J. H. (1989). The somatic sensory system. In J. H. Martin (Ed.), *Neuroanatomy: Text and atlas* (pp. 122-123). New York, NY: Elsevier.

Miller, A. J. (1982). Deglutition. *Physiological Review*, *62*, 129-184.

Robbins, J., & Leviue, R.L. (1988). Swallowing after unilateral stroke of the cerebral cortex: Preliminary experience. *Dysphagia, 3,* 11–17.

Rosenbek, J. C., & Jones H. N. (2009). *Dysphagia in movement disorders.* San Diego, CA: Plural.

Suzuki, M., Asada, Y., Ito, J., Hayashi, K, Inoue, H., & Kitano, H. (2003). Activation of cerebellum and basal ganglia on volitional swallowing detected by functional magnetic resonance imaging. *Dysphagia, 18,* 71–77.

Zald, D. H., & Pardo, J. V. (1999). The functional neuroanatomy of voluntary swallowing. *Annals of Neurology, 46,* 281–286.

4 Clinical Swallowing Examination

The clinical swallow examination (CSE) provides the basis for determining appropriate interventions and recommendations, as well as determining the need for further instrumental assessment. The CSE is but one tool in the clinician's assessment toolbox. Instrumental assessment procedures such as a videofluoroscopic swallow study, a fiberoptic endoscopic swallowing examination, and manometry have important roles, but have limitations with regard to the determination of neuromuscular status (see Chapter 6, Instrumental Examinations). For example, although dynamic radiographic images yield the clearest and most reliable data relative to the biomechanics of swallowing, their data alone are insufficient to make a determination regarding the underlying neuromuscular mechanism.

This chapter focuses on the conceptual framework of the CSE. The CSE is not a procedure that can be implemented by a technician. It requires a level of consistency in making clinical judgments of numerous factors that influence both pathology and function. Quality judgments come from critical analysis of clinical observations within the context of facts and clues provided in the medical record. The attainment of competency in this regard requires extensive experience, repetition of learned techniques, and mentoring, with the goal of developing consistent and effective techniques.

The CSE typically includes three components (Yorkson, Miller, & Strand, 2004):

1. *History:* Obtain information through medical records review and interview regarding diagnosis, prior medical history, background, current speech and swallowing symptoms, management of symptoms, treatment expectations and goals.
2. *Physical/Oral Mechanism Examination:* Evaluate the structure and physiologic function of muscles for speech and swallowing. Observe ancillary signs of physical function that provide additional clues for swallowing function.
3. *Assessment of Swallowing Function:* Evaluate functional swallow ability, risk of aspiration pneumonia or pulmonary complications, ability to maintain adequate nutrition and hydration, secretion management, endurance, and comfort with swallowing.

THE SCIENCE AND ART OF THE PHYSICAL EXAMINATION

The quality of a physical exam is a function of the knowledge and skill of the clinician. When there is no knowledge of specific clinical signs, they will not be elicited from the patient nor recorded by the clinician. DeGowin's classic textbook on the medical diagnostic examination (LeBlond, Brown, & DeGowin, 2009), describes the physical examination by declaring: "Among the examination methods, inspection is the least mechanical and hardest to learn" (p.35). In making the point that an effective examination is dependent on the examiner's knowledge and skill, the authors site the maxims of Maxwell Wintrobe, *"We see what's behind the eyes,"* and Goethe, *"Was man weiss, man sieht"* (What one knows, one sees"). The authors conclude this point by noting, " . . . *sight is a faculty, whereas seeing is an art."* In our view, these writers' description of the physical examination is apropos to the clinical examination for swallowing.

Any conclusion made from a clinical examination is not derived from the sum total of scores based on objective ratings. The product of a clinical examination comes from an analysis of all findings, determining what is significant and what is not, within the balanced context of the clinician's background of knowledge and the patient's unique presentation and circumstance. It requires professional skill, patience, intellectual curiosity, and the ability to reason. To a great extent a full examination requires the cooperation of the patient, although in many instances this is not possible and conclusions will be based on general observations, partial examination data, and deductive reasoning. Finally, the CSE does not purport to be a definitive procedure in the determination of aspiration. Although in many instances even a cursory clinical exam will provide a clinician with sufficient data to be confident in their supposition that an individual is or is not aspirating

when swallowing, there is no objective visualization of the event provided in this procedure. Clinicians have attempted to use various adjuncts to the clinical examination to correlate aspiration with clinical signs, for example, auscultation and monitoring oxygen saturation, but no reliable technique has been developed. However, given the expense and potential discomfort associated with various means of instrumental evaluation, care should be taken in determining necessity for and type of instrumental methods to augment the CSE. A general rule in determining the necessity of additional expensive and/or invasive instrumental examination(s) is to consider whether the results will affect recommendations based on the clinical exam. For instance, if significant risk factors for aspiration are observed during the CSE, confirmation of such factors via an instrumental study likely will not alter recommendations or management of the problems. A related consideration in progressive neurologic disease is timing for instrumental evaluations. For instance, repeated videofluoroscopic swallow studies (VFSS) to track swallowing changes associated with disease progression would result in repeated exposure to radiation and ingestion of barium that potentially could have detrimental side effects.

CSE observations must be considered within the context of the individual's overall risk for aspiration pneumonia, as risk for aspiration pneumonia is not solely related to aspiration of food and/or liquid during eating (Langmore et al., 1998). Other risk factors for aspiration pneumonia include dependency on others for feeding, poor oral hygiene, dental decay, respiratory impairments, an immunocompromised health status, smoking, and impaired pulmonary clearance (Hadjikoutis & Wiles, 2001; Langmore et al., 1998).

There are three important premises that need to be acknowledged relative to the interpretation of data derived from a clinical examination: (1) simultaneous judgments are made of both pathology and function; (2) findings are interpreted in light of one's knowledge of neurologic systems; and (3) no one sign defines the disease or condition.

With regard to judging pathology and function, a skilled examiner initially will determine the degree to which each observation conforms to a theoretical norm. This applies to judgments of structural integrity, the presence of any lesion or abnormal tissue finding, sensory modalities, and the significance of sensory-motor reflexes. Judgments of function require observations of mobile structures and the assessment of several dimensions: stability of the structure at rest, range of motion, speed, precision, strength (force and endurance), timing (coordination or meter), and comparisons of voluntary to involuntary movements.

The findings from a clinical examination should be compared with what is known about the underlying neurologic system(s), both normal and disordered patterns of functioning. For example, at the level of neurons, the nervous system is capable of either excitation or inhibition. Normal movement reflects the balance of excitatory and inhibitory impulses, while abnormalities represent imbalances. Simply put, neuromuscular impairments of spasticity and rigidity reflect errors in inhibitory control at some level, whereas flaccid muscle impairments suggest inadequate excitation or activation of involved muscles. The examiner's task is to correlate data derived from

the inspection and, utilizing the preponderance of evidence, develop a neurologically sound and logical description of the functioning system.

A *pathognomonic* finding means that a single sign or symptom defines a disease. In clinical examination, this can be problematic and one should avoid jumping to conclusions based on any single finding or observation. The systematic recording and analysis of all data should be used to formulate a final assessment.

The tables in this chapter outline the components of the clinical examination across three domains: clinical observations, general physical findings, and focused head and neck examination. Experience completing the examination in total will allow for the development of efficiencies, but the clinician should not sacrifice accuracy and thoroughness for expedience. The sequence of the examination must be adapted to the setting and circumstances, for example, bedside or clinic. With experience, and ideally supported by mentoring, each clinician will refine techniques to facilitate their own inspection and will learn to expand on the examination to augment their data.

The overall process should be viewed as a systematic yet dynamic exercise consisting of a multitude of observations, hypotheses, and analyses of data, leading to further focused inspections and reanalysis. Each observation is an impression or description of what is seen, heard, felt, or smelled; it is not expressed in diagnostic terms or given a label as to its etiology. In the end, the clinician will determine which observations are relevant, that is, the findings fit a recognizable pattern, and which are not applicable to the final assessment. In some cases conclusions will be based on presumptive evidence or circumstances in which one item of data can be presumed based on other highly correlated observations, for example, the patient who drives from work to arrive at an appointment on time can be presumed to be fully oriented at that moment.

Patient History

Knowledge of the primary medical diagnosis and approximate onset date is essential in the evaluation and determination of appropriate intervention. It is not only diagnosis of a particular disease that is needed, but also a determination of the neuromuscular state that is a consequence of that disease. Understanding how specific neuromuscular states affect the swallowing mechanism is critical. Diagnosis influences the rate and pattern of symptom progression and, to some extent, the severity of the impairment, all of which relate to the overall prognosis. Neuromuscular status also influences decisions about which interventions could potentially aid swallowing function.

A review of medical history is essential whether or not a patient has a specific medical diagnosis that is related to a neuromuscular disease. Clinicians should review and obtain data relating to the following domains:

- General health (including the patient's level of independence)
- Family history (pertinent to any inherited diseases or conditions)
- Previous examinations relevant to swallowing or the digestive tract
- Neurologic conditions
- Pulmonary history including current and prior respiratory function, previous episodes of aspiration pneumonia (See further information on this topic in Chapter 5)
- Surgeries pertinent to swallowing and/or the digestive tract
- Psychiatric/psychological health and history
- Interventions relevant to swallowing (head, neck, thorax radiation therapy; esophageal dilation; fundoplication)
- Social history.

The database pertinent to swallowing should include a list of medications that might have an impact. For example, many medications will affect saliva consistency, even causing a dry mouth. Others will affect levels of arousal, energy, ability to concentrate, or behavior. The list of medications should include both current and past medications, and those that have been prescribed or taken over-the-counter.

Equally important in the review of the medical record is the patient's subjective report of their experience with eating and swallowing. Although ideally obtained directly from the patient, often family or other observers will be the source of critical information. At minimum clinicians will want to know: the duration of any problem swallowing, the frequency with which a particular symptom is experienced, and whether the problem is intermittent or constant. Commonly, patients will specify problematic bolus consistencies (e.g., liquids, semisolids, solids); this should be explored in enough detail to allow the examiner to provide specific examples of boluses that present problems. Additionally, note should be made of circumstances that either exacerbate a problem (e.g., "I choke when I am fatigued.") or relieve the difficulty (e.g., "I do well when I'm rested.").

There are questions that should be asked of patients to explore symptoms that are frequently associated with dysphagia. These include the following:

- Do you have any sensation of obstruction? (If yes, specify the location.)
- Is there pain or discomfort associated with swallowing? (If yes, specify site.)
- Does food or liquid [make you choke, cause coughing, go the wrong way]?
- Do you have heartburn or symptoms associated with acid in the throat? (Rule out symptoms associated with laryngopharyngeal reflux [LPR], such as chronic hoarseness, throat clearing, cough, "lump" in throat sensation, excessive mucus or phlegm, metallic taste or other unpleasant tastes, ear pain, and so forth.)
- Have you (or others) noted any unusual mouth odor?
- Does food or liquid ever leak from your nose?

In addition to the above associated symptoms, there are other signs ancillary to the development of dysphagia. These factors are a consequence of impaired swallowing and help to measure the severity of the problem:

- Weight loss (or gain)
- Change in eating habits (where food is eaten, length of time required to eat, foods avoided)
- Change in appetite
- Change in enjoyment of eating
- Altered taste and/or smell sensation
- Saliva change (dry mouth, thickened secretions, excessive saliva)
- Sleep disturbance

- Signs or symptoms of possible aspiration pneumonia (e.g., fever, chest congestion, etc.).

It is critical that examiners observe and inquire about speech functions, as this motor behavior is highly related to swallowing. Although there are major differences with regard to neurologic organization and the demands placed on the musculature, many of the same structures and muscles are common to both functions. Asking the patient, family or other close observer to describe any changes that have been detected in speech is critical.

Clinical Observations

A well-known maxim regarding the art of examination, attributed to the pulmonologist R. Waring, states, *"The examination does not wait the removal of the shirt."* Truly, first impressions are critically important and with practice a clinician can develop more acuity by attending to features of each patient's appearance, affect, behavior, and manner of interaction. The number of data points that can be recorded under clinical observations is ever expanding. In most instances when we encounter a new patient we have an immediate impression—assumptions that are based largely on unconscious observations. Impressions can range from "alert, cooperative, pleasant, fully oriented, healthy appearing . . . " to "agitated, uncooperative, distressed, cachectic appearing . . . " The accuracy of one's initial impression will only become apparent after additional data are obtained and analyzed; but first impressions should not be ignored. Skillful clinicians will learn to recognize the specific behaviors and characteristics that contributed to their impression, and will develop techniques to confirm, modify or reject their initial hypothesis. Table 4–1 lists examples of domains upon which clinicians can focus their attention to help form a reliable clinical impression. These observations serve only as the starting point in the clinical examination, but their importance should not be minimized.

Certainly, the most complex observable human behavior with regard to the demands on the neurologic system is speech and language. Speech alone is the most demanding motor act with regard to the number of muscles involved, the requirements for speed and precision of movement, and the coordination of multiple systems working together. Language involves more than a selection of symbols and the utilization of learned rules of syntax; its full expression draws upon thought, judgment and emotion. Those who are adept at analyzing a patient's speech and language possess a precious talent and have discovered a fruitful vein of data that can be utilized to aid formulation of clinical impressions.

General Physical Findings

"The trouble with most doctors isn't so much that they don't know enough, as it is that they don't see enough." This quote, attributed to the 19th century Irish physician, Sir Dominic Corrigan, is apro-

Table 4–1. Components of the Clinical Exam: Informal Observations

Clinical Observations (Examples)	Examples of Data
Level of alertness	Alert, interactive, somnolent, drowsy, lethargic
Behavior	Appropriate, cooperative, restless, impulsive
Appearance	Appropriate, disheveled, unkempt, older than chronologic age, odor
Attitude	Cooperative or uncooperative, hostile, guarded, suspicious . . .
Affect	Appearing relaxed, anxious, distressed, labile, flat, dysphoric
Nutritional state	Well or undernourished, obese, emaciated
Motor speech	Intelligibility judgment, articulation (rate, precision), resonance, phonation, prosody
Language	Auditory and reading comprehension, spoken and written expression
Mental status	Oriented/disoriented, confused, agitated, drowsy
Level of personal independence	Fully independent, independent with aids, totally or partially dependent (specify area)
Hydration	Well-hydrated, tenting skin, dry mucosa, thick secretions
Medical/Health aids	Hearing aid(s), glasses, PEG, NG, trach tube, prosthesis

pos to the notion that we must observe "outside the box." In this case, the observations cannot be limited to the box that is swallowing, but should extend to the entire physical being of the patient. Obviously, some systems are more relevant than others and reflect data that are pertinent to the patient's ability to swallow. In Table 4-2 examples of anatomic and physiologic systems are outlined, including those that are either inextricably related to swallowing (e.g., respiration), have commonalities with regard to signs of impairment (e.g., skeletal musculature), or, when inspected, can yield information that might be important and relevant to swallowing (e.g., visual system). Whether a clinician

administers specific tests to observe and assess structure and function in these systems, or has learned to interpret findings that have been recorded by specialists who have performed the tests, is not critical. However, based on our experience, attention to these ancillary systems facilitates insight into potential neurologic and/or other physical system dysfunction(s) that might be affecting swallowing.

Focused Head and Neck Examination (Table 4–3)

The ability to interpret findings from a clinical examination is a product of

Table 4–2. Components of the Clinical Exam: General Physical Findings

General Physical Findings (Examples)	Examples of Data
Respiration	Regular, rapid respiratory rate, shallow, clavicular breathing, congested, wheezing, stridor
Voice	Quality (e.g., normal, hoarse, breathy, aphonic), volume, prosody, etc.
Speech	Intelligibility judgment, articulation (rate, precision), resonance, etc.
Skeletal musculature	Atrophy (specify muscles), fasciculations, contractures (specify joints)
UE/LE extremity strength	Hemiplegia, hemiparesis, paraplegia, tetraplegia
Coordination	Overshooting, intention tremor, clumsy, shaky, dysmetria
Muscle and body stability	Tremor (described), involuntary movements, unstable standing and/or sitting
Ambulation	Normal gait, walks with cane, wide-based gait, hemiplegic gait, independent in wheelchair
Visual system	Vacant stare, spontaneous nystagmus, disconjugate gaze (strabismus), visual field impairment (specify quadrant), blindness (one eye or both)
Auditory system	Hearing loss, deafness

Table 4–3. Components of the Clinical Exam: Focused Head and Neck Examination

Head and Neck Findings (Domains)	Data Points
Sensory	Touch and temperature in face (orbital, maxillary, mandibular areas) and oral cavity
Muscles of mastication	Palpate masseter and temporalis in biting/clenching
	Palpate jaw in lateral movement (internal/external pterygoids)
Muscles of facial expression	Observe symmetry at rest, voluntary movement, emotional expression
	Lips: symmetry; palpate in lip seal and retraction
	Platysma: symmetry
	Orbicularis oculi: symmetry
	Frontalis: symmetry
	Note any involuntary movement (fasciculations, tremor, spasming, dyskinesia, myokymia, synkinesis)
Frontal release reflexes	Elicit by tapping: suck, snout
	Observe bite reflex
	May elicit other reflexes (e.g., palmomental, glabellar, grasp)
Intraoral inspection	Mucosa: describe lesions (e.g., erythematous, white, exophytic, ulcerative), saliva consistency
	Teeth/gums: describe overall condition
	Hard palate: shape
	Velum: symmetry at rest, position in oral and nasal breathing, movement on phonation (sustained/unsustained, complete/incomplete) and gag
	Pharyngeal wall: movement on phonation and gag
	Gag reflex: symmetry/completeness of movement (asymmetric, absent, hypoactive, hyperactive)
	Tongue
	Appearance at rest
	Movement: protrusion, palpation/resistance in each cheek, ROM
Larynx	Extrinsic: palpation of elevation on dry swallow
	Intrinsic: inspection (with description of mucosa, structures at rest, symmetry of vocal fold movement, description of observed lesions)
Swallowing	Description of observations during dry swallows and swallows with safe boluses

the quality of one's original preparation, continued guidance, and the amount of experience one has in administering examinations. It is both a science and an art; with nurturing and practice, talent emerges. Even the most talented examiners will need to continuously refine and expand their skills and powers of observation. There is no single sequence or circumscribed set of observations that fit all settings. What follows should be viewed as general guidelines.

Sensory

The trigeminal nerve (CN V) carries somatic senses from the face in three branches: ophthalmic, maxillary, and mandibular (Figure 4–1). It also serves the anterior two-thirds of the oral cavity for touch, pressure and temperature (but not taste). Testing is done on each side of the face in all three divisions with a

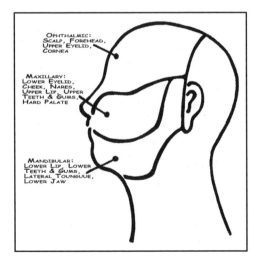

Figure 4–1. Sensory branches of the trigeminal nerve. As depicted, three branches of the trigeminal nerve (Vth CN), the ophthalmic, maxillary, and mandibular, serve somatosensory modalities in the regions of the forehead, midface, and lower jaw.

tissue paper or cotton wisp: forehead, cheeks and chin. The examiner should avoid the lateral mandible as SN C2 and C3 innervate this. Oral mucosa is also tested on both sides.

Although the swallowing exam could be extended to include the sensory modalities of temperature and pain, these data typically are not as useful. However, being able to interpret the results of a neurologist's exam can be extremely helpful. In particular, the corneal reflex frequently is examined and one should know that this test elicits an eye blink by touching each cornea in turn with a cotton wisp, testing sensory V and motor VII.

Taste typically is not tested in the neurologic examination; however, in some cases a clinician will want to include it in the clinical swallowing exam. The anterior two-thirds of the oral cavity (tongue, hard and soft palates) is served by CN VII, the posterior one-third by CNs IX and X. Using solutions of salty, sour, bitter, and sweet flavors, the anterior and posterior tongue are tested, one side at a time. To avoid having the solution move around in the mouth, the examiner should apply a saturated applicator to a specific location on the protruded tongue and have the patient point to the word that represents the taste. The mouth is rinsed between tests.

Because smell is intimately related to taste, olfactory sense may also be tested. Using nonirritating stimulants like cloves, coffee, soap, or perfume, the subject is tested one nostril at a time with the opposite nostril occluded.

Muscles of Mastication

The jaw muscles include: (1) the masseter, a pair of superficial muscles attached superiorly to zygoma and inferiorly to the lateral mandible; (2) the temporalis, a pair of large, flat, superficial muscles lying in the temporal fossa; and (3) the paired internal (medial) and external (lateral) pterygoids that insert into the medial surface of the mandible. The masseter and temporalis muscles, working with the medical pterygoids, are the biting muscles and can exert a compression force greater than any other muscles in the body. They are best assessed by palpation. With the examiner's fingers placed over the temples (temporalis muscles) and above the angle of the mandible (masseter muscles), the patient is asked to bite or clench the jaw (Figure 4–2A). Bulging of the muscles and the functional force of the bite is judged. Given that

these muscles are capable of generating a tremendous degree of force, resistive maneuvers should be avoided because of the risk for temporal-mandibular joint dislocation. The external pterygoid muscles contract to open the jaw, and along with the internal pterygoids provide for lateral jaw movement and participate in the grinding action necessary for chewing. As illustrated in Figure 4–2B, gentle palpation of lateral jaw movement will assess both strength and symmetry. All muscles of mastication are innervated by the trigeminal nerve (CN V).

As part of the inspection of the jaw, judgments of opening should be made. Asymmetries observed at rest and during opening should be noted, but are not

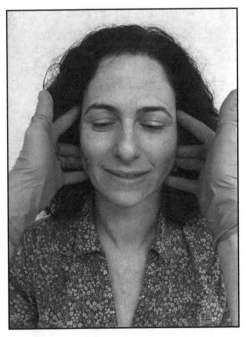 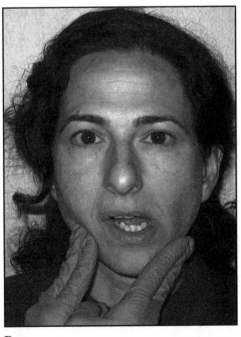

A   **B**

Figure 4–2. Palpating muscles of mastication. By placing the fingers over the temporalis and masseter muscles (**A**) as the patient alternately opens and clenches the jaw the clinician can appreciate the functional strength of these biting muscles. Additionally, gentle palpation of the mandible as the patient moves the jaw side-to-side (**B**) provides information regarding the integrity of the pterygoid muscles.

specific to any neuromuscular problem. Trismus, a limitation in mouth opening, has many potential causes, for example: postradiation therapy, inflammation of muscles of mastication or tissue around the molars, temporal-mandibular joint disorder (TMJ) or TMJ ankylosis, pharyngeal abscess, condylar fracture, brainstem injury, or jaw trauma (Jelasic & Freitag, 1978; Schwerdtfeger & Jelasic, 1985).

Muscles of Facial Expression

Muscles of the face are examined both at rest and during active movement for evidence of asymmetry. At rest, one should observe for the widening of the palpebral fissure (space or opening between the upper and lower eyelids) and/or flattening of the nasolabial fold on one side. Although it is well within normal limits to have some facial asymmetry at rest, movements should be performed symmetrically. Patients should be directed to wrinkle their forehead by frowning and lifting their eyebrows. Testing may include having the patient close their eyes tightly, grimace, or show their teeth and puff out their cheeks while tightly holding their lips closed. In each of these actions, the examiner compares the two sides of the face for symmetry of contraction and overall force. The ability to seal the lips is functionally important to swallowing. In cases where the lower motor neuron (LMN) is impaired anywhere from its origin in the nucleus of the brainstem through the axons of CN VII itself, and including the neuromuscular junction, a lesion will result in complete unilateral facial weakness. This impairment, often referred to as *peripheral facial nerve palsy*, includes the muscles of the forehead (the frontalis) as well as the lower two-thirds of the face (Figure 4–3A). When

only the lower two-thirds of the face is weak (Figure 4–3B), the impairment is referred to as *central facial weakness* and is associated with upper motor neuron (UMN) impairment. The discrepancy between peripheral and central weakness is due to the fact that the muscles of the forehead are fully represented in the motor cortex of both hemispheres. Another observation that will help to differentiate LMN from UMN lesions is found during emotional expression, for example, laughter. When unilateral weakness is due to a LMN lesion, movement on the impaired side is the same for both voluntary and emotional expression, for example. However, when the weakness is related to an UMN lesion, movement is considerably better during emotional expression than during volitional acts (Figure 4–4).

Throughout the inspection of facial muscles examiners should observe for any involuntary movements. Fasciculations around the lips and mentalis (chin) muscles, hemifacial spasming, dyskinetic movements, myokymia (e.g., blephrospasm), or synkinesis (an involuntary movement occurring simultaneously with a voluntary action) may be significant findings.

Frontal Release Reflexes

There are a number of frontal release reflexes that are considered to be either "primitive" or "regressive" reflexes. That is, they are signs that the inhibitory centers located in the frontal lobes bilaterally are not exerting influence on the motor system; thus reflexes that were once present during infancy and later suppressed during nervous system maturation have reappeared as a result of CNS disease. For those patients with impaired inhibitory function, some of these reflexes,

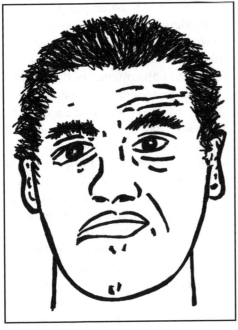
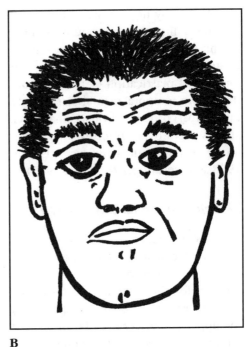

A   **B**

Figure 4–3. Lower motor neuron and upper motor neuron facial weakness.
Unilateral facial weakness due to a LMN impairment (**A**) results in significant weakness
of all facial muscles including *frontalis* muscles of the forehead, *orbicularis oculi* muscle around eye, and the muscles of facial expression in the lower two-thirds of the face.
Because of the complete bilateral representation of the frontalis muscles, in UMN impairment (**B**) the forehead is not impaired and only the lower two-thirds of the face are
weakened and usually to a lesser degree than with LMN involvement.

like the sucking, snouting, biting, and
rooting can be elicited by lightly tapping
the lips, touching the chin, or brushing
the perioral area. In extreme cases the
signs may appear merely by approaching
the mouth with a tongue blade. Other
signs that are considered to be indicators
of impaired inhibitory control are the
glabellar reflex (failure to inhibit an eye
blink when lightly and repeatedly tapped
in the space between the eyebrows), the
grasp reflex (inability to release a grasp
when an object is placed in the palm of
the hand), and the palmomental reflex
(contraction of the ipsilateral mentalis
muscle over the chin when a firm stimu-

lus is drawn diagonally across the palm
of the hand from the wrist up to the base
of thumb). Examiners should be careful
not to overinterpret these signs; however,
positive findings may support one's clinical impression of motor disinhibition.

Intraoral Inspection

There is much that can be appreciated
during inspection of the oral cavity. With
regard to the mucosa, any abnormalities
in appearance should be noted and possibly referred for specific diagnosis. Particularly, lesions that are erythematous
(reddened), white, exophytic (raised or

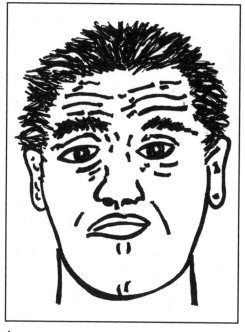

A

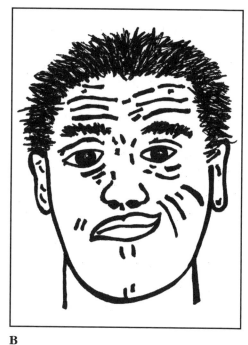

B

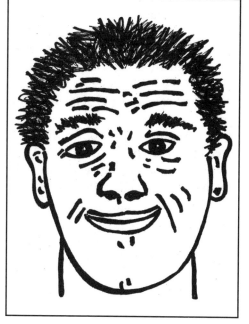

C

Figure 4–4. Muscles of facial expression in UMN impairment. Right-sided weakness is apparent at rest (**A**) with flattening of the nasolabial fold and widening of the palpebral fissure. During voluntary retraction of the lips (**B**) there is asymmetry in movement, however, during emotional expression of a smile (**C**) the movement is much more symmetric.

growing outward), or ulcerative (an open sore) should be considered suspicious. The mucosa should be moist, but conditions like dryness or excessive saliva should be noted. Observing the condition of the teeth and gums is important,

as is observing of the shape of the hard palate and velum at rest. With regard to the velum, asymmetry with the uvula pulled to one side suggests weakness on the opposite side. Observing movement of the velum during quiet breathing, forced oral and nasal breathing, and during phonation is important.

A gag reflex can be elicited from many points in the oral cavity. Some individuals will display strong contractions of the velum and pharyngeal wall with little or no touch stimulation, whereas others will not gag even after strong and repeated stimulation in the posterior oral cavity. The variability of gag in normal subjects makes this reflex particularly difficult to interpret. As a general guideline, we recommend the following considerations: (1) a gag that is judged to be hyperactive is only significant when it is accompanied by other signs that suggest impaired motor inhibition, usually associated with bilateral upper motor neuron impairment, for example, dysarthria with spastic features, frontal release signs, cognitive impairments and emotional lability; (2) a gag that is hypoactive or absent is significant only when it is accompanied by other indicators for lower motor neuron or bulbar impairment, for example, loss of sensation in the posterior oral cavity, dysarthria with flaccid features like hypernasality with nasal air loss, and dysphagia with nasal regurgitation; and (3) an asymmetrical gag, in which movement can be elicited only by stimulation on one side or when only one side contracts, is suggestive of an ipsilateral brainstem or peripheral nerve lesion. Figure 4–5 illustrates the neurologic systems involved in the sensory-motor gag reflex and indicate what happens with lesions at various levels of the system.

Tongue function is critical to swallowing. At rest the tongue should appear symmetrical in bulk and without excessive spontaneous movement. Observations of atrophy and fasciculations often suggest LMN impairment. UMN lesions, when bilateral, lead to spasticity and concomitant slowing of movements. Inability or hesitation in performing voluntary movements of the tongue, such as protrusion and lateralization, may suggest an oral apraxia. Deviation of the tongue from the midline during protrusion is interpreted as unilateral weakness on the side to which it deviates. In effect, as the tongue pushes outward, the stronger side deflects the tongue toward the weaker side. With a LMN lesion or injury, deviation of the tongue will occur toward the same side as the lesion; with an UMN lesion or injury, the tongue will deviate to the contralateral side (Figure 4–6). Having the patient push the tongue into each cheek while the examiner resists the movement is an effective method of assessing lingual strength and range of motion (ROM). Speed, quickness, and control are assessed during isolated, rapid lateral movements of the tongue or by rapid forward-back movements. These features can also be evaluated during the patient's performance of diadochokinetic speech tasks (e.g., tah-tah-tah. . .). Objective measures of tongue strength can be obtained by employing an Iowa Oral Pressure Instrument (IOPI).

Laryngeal Examination

When an examiner palpates the larynx as the patient swallows, there is an opportunity to subjectively judge the strength, timing and completeness of an essential component in oral-pharyngeal swallow-

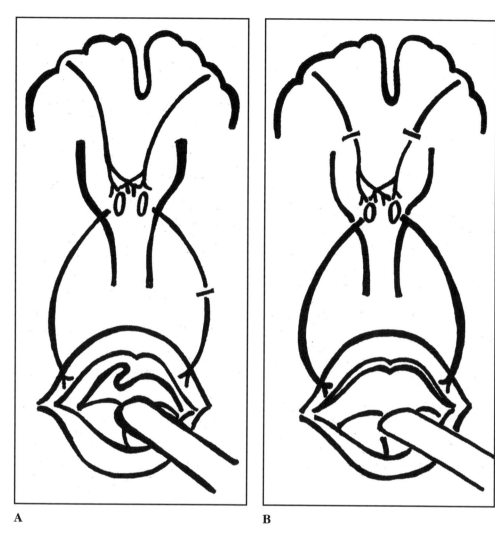

A   B

Figure 4–5. Levels of impairment affecting the gag reflex. In cases with unilateral LMN lesions as depicted here (**A**), the velar and pharyngeal contractions are asymmetric and diminished to absent on the impaired left side and the uvula is pulled toward the stronger right side. With bilateral UMN lesions (**B**), there is a loss of inhibitory influence on the gag reflex and it tends to be hyperactive.

ing. To assess laryngeal ascent, the examiner's index finger is typically placed with gentle pressure between the hyoid bone and thyroid cartilage at the thyroid notch as illustrated in Figure 4-7. Elevation of the larynx is critical to epiglottic inversion and protection of the laryngeal entrance, cessation of breathing, channeling of a bolus away from the airway, and mechanical pull exerted on the posterior cricopharyngeal muscle that is necessary for opening the upper esophageal sphincter (UES). The anterior-superior movement of the larynx is a product of

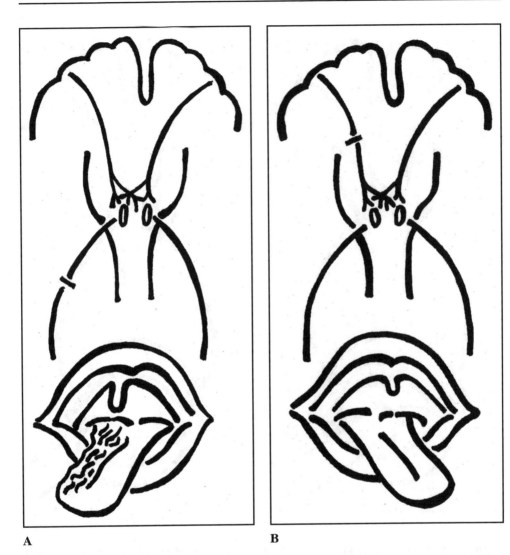

A   B

Figure 4–6. Levels of impairment affecting the tongue. A complete unilateral LMN lesion as depicted here on the right side (**A**) will result in right-sided lingual weakness with atrophic findings that may include visible fasciculations. When a unilateral UMN lesion affects tongue strength, as depicted here in the right hemisphere (**B**), contralateral weakness is expected. Note that on protrusion of the tongue, there is deviation toward the weaker side and the deviation is more pronounced in cases with LMN impairment.

an exquisite sequence of muscle contractions primarily involving extrinsic laryngeal muscles attached to the hyoid bone. The examiner's assessment of this particular muscle action is often a critical piece of the overall clinical swallowing evaluation, yet the quality of the data is based on the examiner's experience and other factors that influence competency.

A clinical examination that includes laryngoscopy will provide important data, yet in our experience this rarely is performed as part of the CSE. This assessment is accomplished using a fiberoptic

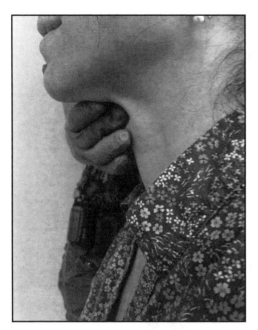

Figure 4–7. Palpation of laryngeal elevation. Placing fingers at the hyoid bone and thyroid cartilage during a swallow will allow a clinician to appreciate the initiation of the pharyngeal stage of swallowing. Judgments of strength, completeness and timing are highly subjective and require a great deal of experience before they become reliable.

scope, either a rigid scope for transoral exam, or flexible scope for nasopharyngeal insertion. Inspection at rest reveals the state of the mucosa (e.g., irritated, inflamed, dry), any pooling in the recesses of the hypopharynx (e.g., in valleculae or piriform sinuses), status of the airway (e.g., congested, clear), and integrity of structures (e.g., symmetric, obstructed). Mobility of the vocal folds can be appreciated on this examination as the patient executes various phonatory and valsalva maneuvers and breathing exercises. Any findings that raise suspicion for a structural and/or functional impairment should be referred for a complete laryngological examination. Figure 4-8 illustrates the structures that typically are visualized on a laryngoscopic examination.

Swallowing

Decisions regarding the feasibility of proceeding to test swallows are based on an analysis of all data gathered to this point during the CSE. In a real sense this equates to *clinical judgment*. Once an examiner has determined that the patient is safe to attempt test swallows, the assessment can proceed beyond dry swallowing. Often, this part of the examination begins by challenging the patient to suck and/or sip liquid boluses to elicit swallowing. Based on the patient's performance here, the test may proceed to the ingestion of semisolid or solid boluses to elicit chewing and oral manipulation. The *clinical judgment* used to determine the relative safety for a given patient to proceed through this part of the assessment is critical. Some of the factors directly related to swallowing function include: (1) the adequacy of the protective cough reflex; (2) related functions of breathing (e.g., congested vs. clear) and voice (e.g., wet vs. dry; breathy vs. strong); (3) the integrity of the sensory system, particularly in the area of the posterior oral cavity and pharyngeal wall; and (4) the timing and force of laryngeal elevation. Additional judgments are made relative to a patient's level of consciousness, cognitive functions, relative degree of independence, and ability to cooperate with an examination and feeding. Perhaps, the most important factor that is used to make a decision to challenge swallowing during a clinical examination is the patient's overall health status. Obviously, a clinician will be more apt to challenge a patient with a variety of bolus consistencies if that patient is generally healthy

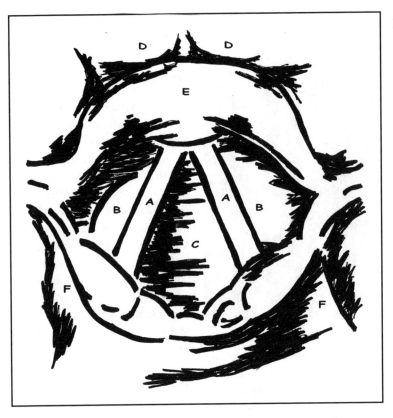

Figure 4–8. Internal laryngeal structures. A thorough inspection of internal laryngeal structures should include (**A**) the true vocal folds, (**B**) the false vocal folds, (**C**) the glottis, (**D**) the valleculae, (**E**) the epiglottis, and (**F**) the piriform sinuses.

and has been eating and drinking prior to the examination.

Determinations regarding how to proceed with test swallows will be made on the basis of the presenting complaints; the symptoms described; what, if anything, is known about the diagnosis; and observations made during the physical examination. Although the specifics of a test swallow depend on the clinical assessment, for most patients it generally is safe to observe swallows using small sips of water and/or a bolus of ice chips. Observations of chewing, oral efficiency, and initiation of swallows provide data relative to the functional integrity of the swallowing mechanism. How the examination proceeds will depend on the information gathered from a patient's first attempts to swallow. Typically, a clinician will progress to solid food boluses and other liquid consistencies in a cautious manner, ensuring the patient's safety as each new bolus consistency is introduced. Clinical signs are not objective indicators of aspiration; therefore, clinicians must rely on their *clinical judgment* to determine the significance of each separate observation and their summative analysis of all data in order to proceed with test swallows. For each swallow attempt the following data should be considered:

- general behavior
  - manner of feeding
  - head turning, head nodding
  - throat clearing
  - oral clearance and/or retention
  - swallow latency
- palpation of laryngeal elevation during an elicited swallow
  - timing of swallow
  - completeness of excursion
- signs of airway compromise
  - change in breathing
  - coughing
  - airway congestion
  - wet voice
- patient's subjective report
  - food sticking (if so, specify locus)
  - sense of airway penetration
  - nasal regurgitation
  - pain or discomfort

The data derived from test swallows are important for the clinician to decide what additional tests are necessary and what steps should be taken to aid the patient who is experiencing difficulties in swallowing. Rarely are the data sufficient to make definitive determinations regarding needed diet adjustments or the effectiveness of particular compensatory swallowing strategies, but observations made during this portion of the CSE are critically important in directing the clinician to ask the appropriate questions that will guide them in completing the full assessment.

CONCLUDING THOUGHTS

From the CSE a clinician should begin to formulate hypotheses regarding the most likely neuromuscular basis for any observed impairment in the swallowing musculature. This does not mean the diagnosis of a specific disease, syndrome, or condition, but rather an understanding of the underlying neuromuscular mechanisms that are influencing function. Furthermore, the CSE should provide important information regarding the functional integrity of the swallowing mechanism. Although it does not allege to prove or disprove the presence or absence of aspiration, as clearly this cannot be visualized or reliably detected from this inspection, there is a determination regarding risk factors for airway penetration and protection. In some cases, aspiration can be presumed to have occurred based on the observed behaviors; in other instances aspiration will be confidently judged to be a remote risk. Frequently, the data obtained during the course of a clinical examination allow clinicians to utilize other assessment tools, for example, fluoroscopy and/or endoscopy, in a more discerning and directed manner. Instrumental assessments are far superior to clinical examinations with regard to the assessment of the biomechanics of swallowing, but only the clinical examination and the analysis of the derivative data can determine the underlying neuromuscular conditions that are contributing to impairment.

REFERENCES

Hadjikoutis, S., & Wiles, C. M. (2001). Respiratory complications related to bulbar dysfunction in motor neuron disease. *Acta Neurologica Scandinavica, 103,* 207–213.

Jelasic, F., & Freitag, V. (1978). Inverse activity of masticatory muscles with and without trismus: A brainstem syndrome. *Journal of Neurology, Neurosurgery and Psychiatry, 41*(9), 798–804.

Langmore, S. E., Terpenning, M. S., Schork, A., Yinmiao, C., Murray, J. T., Lopatin, D., . . . Loesche, W. J. (1998). Predictors of aspiration pneumonia: How important is dysphagia? *Dysphagia, 13,* 69–81.

LeBlond, R. F., Brown, D. D., & DeGowin, R. L. (2009). *DeGowin's diagnostic examination* (9th ed.). New York, NY: McGraw-Hill.

Schwerdtfeger, K., & Jelasic, F. (1985). Trismus in postoperative, posttraumatic and other brain stem lesions caused by paradoxical activity of masticatory muscles. *Acta Neurochirurgica, 76*(1–2), 62–66.

Yorkson, K. M., Miller, B. M., & Strand, E. A. (2004). *Management of speech and swallowing in degenerative diseases* (2nd ed.). Austin, TX: Pro-Ed.

5 Respiratory System and Examination

A key goal of any swallowing evaluation is to assess one's risk for aspiration pneumonia. However, dysphagia is not the sole factor to consider in determining an individual's risk for aspiration pneumonia. Dysphagia and aspiration have been consistently associated with aspiration pneumonia (Langmore et al., 1998). However, factors such as dependency for feeding and/or oral care, number of decayed teeth, tube feeding, multiple (≥1) diagnoses, number of medications and smoking have been shown to be better independent predictors of aspiration pneumonia than dysphagia (Langmore et al., 1998). Factors associated with aspiration pneumonia include dysphagia (with and without aspiration), but also include other factors, for example, chronic obstructive pulmonary disease (COPD), gastrointestinal (GI) disease, poor secretion management, reduced esophageal motility, dental disease, poor oral care, and tube feeding (Langmore et al., 1998). Therefore, consideration of respiratory function, pulmonary defenses and background medical information is vital to evaluation and treatment of swallowing. Signs and symptoms observed during a swallowing evaluation must be considered within the context of the individual's overall risk for aspiration pneumonia, as risk for aspiration pneumonia is not solely related to aspiration (Langmore et al., 1998). For these reasons, this chapter reviews the basics of respiratory anatomy and physiology, pulmonary defenses, and assessment of respiratory function. These topics are discussed within the context of relevance to swallowing and risk for aspiration pneumonia.

RESPIRATORY ANATOMY AND PHYSIOLOGY

Many of the same anatomic structures used for swallowing and speech are needed for breathing. Basic respiratory system anatomy is illustrated in Figure 5–1. The larynx separates the upper and lower respiratory systems. As the trachea descends it bifurcates into two bronchi at the main laryngeal carina. From there it continues to bifurcate in the lung 22 to 23 times until it reaches the level of the alveoli. At the alveolar level, the surface area of the lung has increased dramatically. The alveoli are wrapped in capillaries to allow for gas exchange to occur across this great surface area. Millions of alveoli make up the bulk of the two lungs in the human body. The right lung has three lobes and contains approximately 55% of the total lung volume. The left lung with two lobes

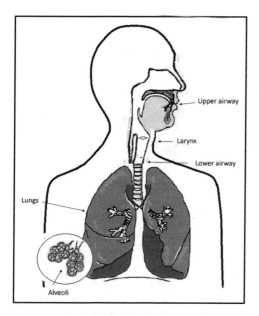

Figure 5–1. Basic respiratory anatomy. The airway begins at the mouth and nose and ends with the lungs. The larynx separates the upper and lower respiratory systems. When air has reached alveoli within the lungs, the surface area has increased dramatically to allow for gas exchange.

is a little smaller than the right owing to space taken by the heart. The lungs are contained within the bony structures of the rib cage, thoracic vertebrae and sternum, collectively referred to as the thorax.

As movement of lung tissue is passive, mechanical and muscular forces are needed to move air in and out. The muscles of the respiratory system can be divided into two groups: *respiratory pump muscles* and *respiratory valve muscles*. The *respiratory pump muscles* include separate muscle groups that aid inspiration versus expiration. Several groups of muscles facilitate air intake by creating negative pressure in the expanding lungs. The diaphragm is the primary muscle of inspiration. It is responsible for approxi-

mately 65% of vital capacity in normally functioning persons. The diaphragm moves downward with contraction, expanding the lungs and thoracic cavity. The external intercostals and accessory muscles further expand the thoracic cage. Expansion of thoracic space creates a negative air pressure within the lungs. Then, in accordance with Boyle's law, air flows from the region of relatively high pressure (in the atmosphere) to the region of relatively low air pressure (the expanded lungs). Expiration during tidal breathing occurs passively as the muscles of inspiration relax. In certain circumstances, such as cough and speech, expiratory muscles aid forced exhalation. The abdominal muscles are the primary support for forceful exhalation. Table 5-1 lists the respiratory muscles that function during inspiration versus expiration.

The *respiratory valve muscles* consist primarily of the intrinsic laryngeal muscles that control vocal fold movements. The vocal folds have important functions related to the regulation of airflow associated with breathing. For instance, they actively abduct (open) to allow airflow in and out. During activities requiring protection of the airway, for example, swallowing or vomiting, the vocal folds and supraglottic structures close to protect the airway. Function of the vocal folds and supraglottic structures during cough is more complex and are described later in this chapter.

The thoracic cage and lungs have mechanical properties that provide a balance of forces. The lungs naturally recoil inward whereas the rib cage naturally recoils outward. Functional residual capacity (FRC) is the air volume within the lungs when these forces are balanced, also known as the resting volume of the

Table 5–1. Respiratory Pump Muscles

Inspiration

- Diaphragm (Phrenic N; C3–5)
- External intercostals (T1–T12)
- Accessory muscles (Cranial N XI through T1)

Expiration

- Abdominals (T6–L1)
- Internal intercostals (T1–T12)

respiratory system (Figure 5-2). Understanding the mechanical concepts of compliance and elasticity are critical to the appreciation of lung function. Lung compliance specifies how easy it is to inflate the lungs. It is known to vary depending on the volume of air in the lungs. Compliance depends on the properties of both the lungs and the thoracic cage. For instance, in idiopathic pulmonary fibrosis, scarring of lung tissue can result in stiffness, which in turn reduces lung compliance. Conversely, lung elasticity, the ability of lung tissues to recoil after being stretched, is determined primarily by the properties of the lung tissue itself. For example, damage to alveolar walls associated with emphysema, an obstructive lung disease, results in reduced recoil of lung tissue. This in turn creates difficulty with achieving adequate exhalation.

Coordination of Respiration and Swallowing

The upper airway serves multifunctional purposes: swallowing, speech, and breathing. Respiratory and swallowing neurons are situated within close proximity in the lower brainstem. Normal breathing is controlled by a central pattern generator (CPG) in the brainstem that integrates and drives the rhythm of breathing, based in part on sensory feedback from the body. However, this continual rhythmic breathing oscillator must accommodate other functions of the upper respiratory tract, including swallowing, while maintaining adequate respiration. The CPG for the rhythm of breathing is in the medulla and has a close functional relationship with the CPG for swallowing. Fundamentally, patterns of coordination between breathing and swallowing can be characterized by the following parameters: (1) swallow apnea, sometimes referred to as a "respiratory pause," a centrally controlled cessation of breathing that occurs during the swallow, and (2) respiratory-phase patterns, that is, the type of respiration that occurs before and after the swallow, inspiration or expiration. These factors occur within the context of a sequenced and coordinated pattern of events that integrate swallowing and respiration. However, as could be expected, there are multiple variables that affect these parameters as well.

Swallow apnea duration (SAD), or the length of respiratory cessation that occurs during a swallow, has been studied extensively across a variety of conditions. In normally functioning people swallowing single sips of water or other thin liquids, SAD is typically within the range of 0.5 to 1.5 seconds (Boden et al., 2009; Martin, Logemann, Shaker, & Dodds, 1994; Martin-Harris, 2008; Martin-Harris et al., 2005; Martin-Harris, Brodsky, Price, Michel, & Walters, 2003; Matsuo & Palmer, 2009; Selley, Flack, Ellis, & Brooks, 1989).

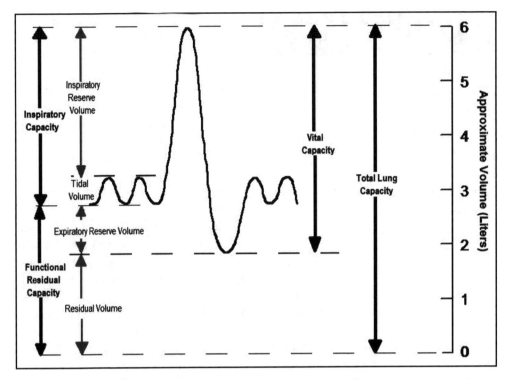

Figure 5–2. Lung volumes and capacities. Lung volumes and capacities are reported in pulmonary function testing and are key to diagnosing many pulmonary conditions. Lung capacities are sums of lung volumes.

VOLUMES:

Tidal volume (TV): Volume of air inspired/expired with normal breathing at rest.

Inspiratory reserve volume (IRV): Maximum volume of air that can be inspired beyond the normal TV.

Expiratory Reserve Volume (ERV): Maximal volume that can be expired beyond the normal TV.

Residual Volume (RV): Volume of air remaining in the lungs after a maximal expiration.

CAPACITIES:

Inspiratory Capacity (IC): TV + IRV
Volume of air inspired with a maximal inspiration.

Functional Residual Capacity (FRC): ERV + RV
Volume of air remaining in lungs following a resting expiration.

Vital Capacity (VC): IRV + TV + ERV = IC + ERV
Volume of air expired with maximal inspiration and expiration.

Total Lung Capacity (TLC): IRV + TV + ERV + RV = IC + FRC
Volume of air in the lungs with a maximal inspiration.

Evidence indicates that the swallow apnea occurs due to central inhibition of respiration, as opposed to obstruction of airflow related to glottic closure only (Matsuo & Palmer, 2009; Nishino & Hiraga, 1991). For instance, respiratory cessation associated with swallowing has been observed in people who are intubated, that is, a breathing tube inserted between the vocal folds that mechanically blocks glottic closure (Nishino & Hiraga, 1991), and people who have undergone laryngectomy (Charbonneau, Lund, & McFarland, 2005; Hiss, Strauss, Treole, Stuart, & Boutilier, 2003).

Martin-Harris (2005) delineated four respiratory-phase patterns that can potentially occur before and after a swallow: expiration/expiration (EX/EX); expiration/inspiration (EX/IN); inspiration/expiration (IN/EX); and, inspiration/inspiration (IN/IN) (Martin-Harris, et al., 2005). Most published studies have examined this relationship during swallows with small amounts of water or other thin liquid boluses, one sip at a time (Matsuo & Palmer, 2009). The most common pattern observed during single sip thin liquid swallowing tasks in normally functioning adults is EX/EX (71–75%), followed by IN/EX (18–22%) (Martin-Harris et al., 2005). This study and many others indicate that expiration occurs after the swallow 95% of the time during single-sip, thin liquid swallowing in normally functioning people (Boden et al., 2009; Hadjikoutis, Pickersgill, Dawson, & Wiles, 2000; Martin et al., 1994; Martin-Harris, 2008; Martin-Harris et al., 2005; Martin-Harris, et al., 2003; Preiksaitis, Mayrand, Robins, & Diamant, 1992; Selley, et al., 1989; Terzi et al., 2007).

Coordination between swallowing and respiration can vary depending on a number of conditions, including volume, viscosity, method to ingestion, body position, and age (Matsuo & Palmer, 2009). For instance, percentages of inspiration before and after swallow apnea are much higher with sequential swallows as opposed to single liquid swallows (Dozier, Brodsky, Michel, Walters, & Martin-Harris, 2006). These patterns may be also altered in the presence of overriding respiratory needs, for example, hypercapnia (elevated levels of carbon dioxide in the blood) (Boden et al., 2009), and/or in the presence of neurologic dysfunction affecting any level, that is, brain, brainstem, spinal cord, and/or peripheral nerve injuries. Certain variables have been shown to have no effect on respiratory-phase patterns or SAD, including sex and race (Dozier et al., 2006; Martin-Harris et al., 2005).

Subglottic Pressure and Swallowing

Gross (2009) reviewed a series of studies examining the significance of subglottic pressure during swallowing, also known as *deglutitive subglottic pressure*. This work initially focused on swallowing efficiency and aspiration risk associated with occluded versus open tracheostomies. With an open tracheostomy, subglottic pressure is always zero, as the air leaks out via the tracheostomy tube. Pressures have been reported to range from 7 to 10 cm H_2O with the tracheostomy tube occluded (Gross, 2009). Although there has been some debate as to the effect of a tracheostomy tube occlusion on aspiration, a majority of studies have revealed associations between tracheostomy tube occlusion and risk for aspiration (Gross, 2009). In one subject without a tracheostomy, a linear relationship was observed between deglutitive subglottic pressure and lung volume (Gross, 2009). Greater speed and efficiency of swallowing has been associated with higher lung volumes. Prolongation of temporal swallowing events has been associated with lower lung volumes (Gross, 2009), leading the investigator to theorize that subglottic pressure might serve as a component of the sensory integration process that links respiration and swallowing CPGs. Terzi et al. (2007) reported an association between maximum inspiratory pressure (MIP) and abnormal coordination of swallowing and breathing. Their subjects included some with nonbulbar neuromuscular disease and capped tracheostomies. In these subjects, swallowing and breathing coordination was improved while patients were on mechanical ventilation. These findings support the potential positive effect of a higher lung volume or increased subglottic pressure on swallowing function.

The Effect of Body Position on Breathing

Respiratory mechanics are affected by body position, as the effects of gravity on the body change in different positions. In supine position the effects of gravity on the contents of the abdomen will push the diaphragm toward the head. Therefore, in normally functioning people, functional residual capacity and vital capacity will be lower in supine position and higher in upright position. These patterns of breathing change in association with shifts in position change in the context of different types of neuromuscular dysfunction. For instance, diaphragm paralysis can result in orthopnea, that is, difficulty breathing in a supine position (Qureshi, 2009). The effect of posture on

breathing is frequently opposite, however, in the context of spinal cord injury (SCI). For instance, complete cervical SCI at C4–C8 results in weakness of the abdominal and intercostal muscles. When seated upright, patients with this form of injury display a paradoxical breathing pattern in which strong diaphragmatic contractions are unopposed by the abdominal and intercostal muscles. This results in lower abdominal distension and upper thoracic collapse during breathing attempts in upright position. In this situation supine position actually aids the ability to take in more air, as the abdominal viscera provides more support due to the pull of gravity (Baydur, Adkins, & Milic-Emili, 2001).

PULMONARY DEFENSES

Normal human pulmonary defenses guard the lungs from infections, such as pneumonia that occurs due to aspiration of food or bacteria and/or inhalation of airborne toxins. These lung defenses include protective anatomic features, airway reflexes, mucocillary clearance, and cellular protections at the level of the alveoli (Happel, Bagby, & Nelson, 2004). Certain anatomic features block entry of larger toxic air particles, liquids and foods to the lungs. For instance, the hairs and turbinates within the nose function as air filters. Other examples include the larger airway protection afforded by reflexive vocal fold closure and epiglottic inversion, as seen during normal swallowing. Airway reflexes, such as sneeze, cough, reflexive swallow, and gag, facilitate expulsion of material that might be toxic to lung tissue. Cellular defenses exist in the larger airways (e.g., the epithelial fluid lining the airways contains antibacterial peptides) and on down to the level of the alveoli (e.g., the alveolar macrophage and other immune system responses). Impairments of the immune system can undermine these defenses (Happel et al., 2004).

Mucociliary clearance, sometimes referred to as the "mucocillary escalator," consists of mucous producing cells and tiny cilia lining the mucosa of the bronchi and bronchioles that beat in a rhythmic fashion to bring up aspirated particles to the larger airways and/or hypopharynx where they can then be swallowed or coughed up and expectorated (Figure 5–3). A fluid layer surrounding the cilia is also needed for normal mucociliary clearance (Finder, 2010). A variety of anti-inflammatory and antimicrobial substances are secreted by epithelial cells to aid the immune response (Bals, Weiner,

& Wilson, 1999). Impairments of mucociliary clearance can occur due to chronic retention of secretions, viral infections, smoking, and ciliary dyskinesia syndromes.

The ability to cough is an essential component of human pulmonary defenses, as cough is one of the most effective means of airway clearance (Happel et al., 2004). An effective cough defends the airway and lungs from aspiration. Cough dysfunction heightens the risk for aspiration pneumonia. This is especially relevant for people with neurologic injury or disease. A protective cough response normally may be initiated volitionally or elicited reflexively when sensory receptors within the mucosa of the larynx and lower airway regions are stimulated (Boitano, 2006). Effective coughing requires an intact cough reflex mechanism, adequate upper airway sensation, as well as adequate respiratory and laryngeal muscle

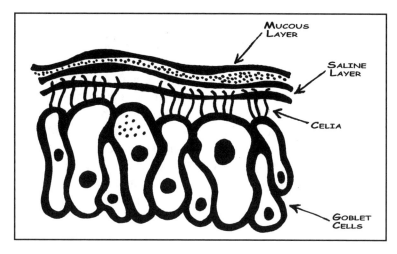

Figure 5–3. Mucociliary clearance. Mucocillary clearance is sometimes referred to as the "mucocillary escalator." Mucous producing goblet cells and rhythmically beating cilia lining the epithelium within the bronchi, bronchioles and nose work in concert to carry mucous up and into the throat, where it can be expectorated or swallowed. Mucocillary clearance is an important component of pulmonary defenses.

strength and coordination. There are at least three sequential phases that facilitate the ability to cough normally (Boitano, 2006): (1) inspiration; (2) compression (intrathoracic pressure build); and (3) expiration (forceful expulsion of air and mucous). It is well known that respiratory muscles are needed for inspiration (e.g., the diaphragm), as well as for the pressure build up necessary for forced expiration (e.g., abdominal muscles). However, vocal fold movements are also integral to cough physiology and occur in sync with these phases (Hillel, 2001; Poletto, Verdun, Strominger, & Ludlow, 2004; von Leden & Isshiki, 1965). During inspiration, the vocal folds abduct (open) to allow airflow to the lungs. Then, both the true vocal folds and supraglottic structures close with contraction of the abdominal muscles to aid in the buildup of intrathoracic air pressure. Vocal fold abduction during expulsion occurs with active contraction of the posterior cricoarytenoid (Hillel, 2001; Poletto et al., 2004); it is not a purely passive response to the force of air pressure. Through electromyography of the laryngeal muscles during cough, Hillel (2001) discovered that the primary laryngeal abductor muscles, that is, posterior cricoarytenoid and cricothyroid, begin to activate (simultaneously with the adductors) just prior to vocal fold abduction during expulsion. This results in an extremely rapid, "spring-load"-like, active abduction of the vocal folds during the expulsion phase (Figure 5–4).

A distinction between reflexively versus volitionally initiated cough is made evident in the literature. A volitional cough is cortically mediated and can be initiated with or without laryngeal sensations or spoken requests (Stephens, Addington, & Widdicombe, 2003). Cough also can be

suppressed volitionally. Conversely, a reflexive cough, or "laryngeal cough reflex," is a brainstem mediated reflex triggered by sensations in the larynx, for example, aspiration of food or liquid (Stephens et al., 2003). Different patterns of motor activation of respiratory muscles have been observed in volitional versus reflexive cough (Lasserson et al., 2006). Muscular activation associated with volitional cough tends to occur more slowly than with reflexive cough, and it is characterized by a graded increase in the activation of expiratory respiratory muscles followed by activation of accessory muscles that is proportional to the cough flow rate. Conversely, reflexive cough is characterized by faster, stronger, and simultaneous activation of expiratory and accessory muscles. In contrast to volitional cough, accessory muscles also show greater activity. Further evidence for a distinction between mechanisms of volitional versus reflexive cough is seen in studies examining "cough apraxia," that is, inability to initiate a cough upon command (Stephens et al., 2003). Stephens et al. (2003) compared volitional and reflexive cough in subjects with right and left middle cerebral artery (MCA) infarcts. Reflexive cough was elicited with inhalation of tartaric acid. Both groups had a normal laryngeal cough reflex. However, 79% of subjects with left MCA infarct demonstrated abnormal volitional cough; 43% of these subjects were unable to initiate and/or sequence the movements associated with volitional cough. This observation was designated as "cough apraxia," or an impaired voluntary cough in the presence of a normal reflexive cough. Subjects with right MCA infarcts demonstrated normal reflexive and volitional coughs. None of these subjects developed aspiration pneumonia. This

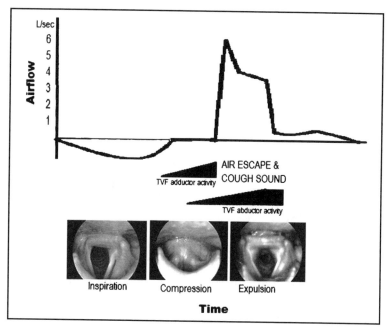

Figure 5–4. Schematic diagram of the vocal fold movements and laryngeal muscle activity during cough. The true vocal folds (TVF) actively abduct during inspiration. During the compression phase of cough, vocal fold closure is reinforced by tight closure of supraglottic structures. During the expulsion phase, the vocal folds actively abduct in concert with the force of airflow through the glottis. Hillel (2001) discovered through EMG of the laryngeal muscles during cough that the primary laryngeal abductor muscles, that is, posterior cricoarytenoid and cricothyroid, begin to activate simultaneously with the primary laryngeal adductor muscles just prior to the expulsion phase of cough. This results in an explosively rapid ("spring-loaded") response of active abduction of the vocal folds during the expulsion phase of cough to forcefully accentuate the rapid flow of air and mucus.

study supports the notion of differential central processing for reflexive versus volitional cough, despite sharing the same efferent motoric sequence. Understanding this concept is important, not only for patients who have experienced a stroke, but also those with degenerative neuromuscular diseases.

Smith-Hammond et al. (2009) asserts that certain volitional cough measures might be more sensitive to detecting risk for aspiration than subjective observations of reflexive cough associated with eating (Smith-Hammond, 2008; Smith-Hammond et al., 2009). Specifically, the cough measures are *expulsive phase rise time, volume acceleration*, and *peak expiratory cough flow* (PECF). Figure 5–5 presents a schematic diagram of these measures. This rationale in part is based on the fact that silent aspiration, that is, aspiration without cough, can occur for

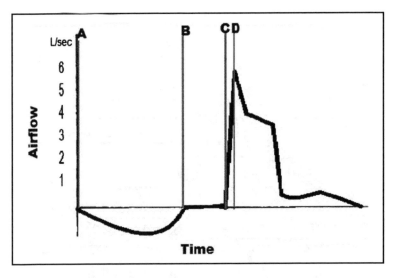

Figure 5–5. Schematic of volitional cough phase measures.

- Inspiratory phase: A to B
- Compression phase: B to C
- Expulsion phase rise time (EPRT): C to D

Measures that have been predictive of aspiration in stroke patients (Smith-Hammond, 2008):

- Expulsion phase rise time (EPRT)
- Peak expiratory cough flow (PECF)
- "Volume acceleration" (VA): PECF / EPRT

some people with neurologic impairments. In studying volitional coughs produced by stroke survivors, *expulsive phase rise time* and *volume acceleration* were independently associated with aspiration risk as determined by scores of ≥5 on the Penetration Aspiration Scale (Smith-Hammond et al., 2009). Volitional cough *expulsion phase rise time* was reported to have 91% sensitivity and 88% specificity in detecting aspiration in stroke survivors (Smith-Hammond, 2008). Volitional cough *volume acceleration* was reported to have 91% sensitivity and 92% specificity in detecting aspiration (as confirmed via instrumental testing) in the same population (Smith-Hammond, 2008). Although norms on these measures currently do not exist, Smith-Hammond et al. 2009, reported that an *expulsive phase rise time* of >67 ms or a *volume acceleration* of <33 mL/s/s identified >90% of aspirators. It is likely that future research will prove that these same indicators are relevant to patients with certain neuromuscular diseases.

Some conditions will compromise normal pulmonary defenses. For instance breathing through a tracheostomy tube will bypass some of the filters that normally protect the lungs, and it can change the ability to build subglottic pressure during cough and swallowing. Various neuromuscular diseases impair muscle strength needed for effective respiration, cough, or swallowing. A variety of pulmonary diagnoses, for example, COPD, can result in higher overall risk for pneumonia. Table 5-2 presents other conditions that might impair one's pulmonary defenses.

What Is Pneumonia?

Failure of pulmonary defenses can result in pneumonia. Pneumonia is an infection in one or both of the lungs. It typically is characterized by inflammation and/or consolidation of the lung parenchyma. Consolidated and/or collapsed lungs lead to shunting that prevents adequate ventilation. A shunt in this context refers to blood that passes from the venous to the arterial system without gas exchange. Since gas is not being exchanged during breathing in this condition, providing additional oxygen to the patient does not help. Signs and symptoms of pneumonia include (but are not limited to) fever, congested coughing, dyspnea, chest pain,

malaise, fatigue, muscle aches, tachycardia, tachypnea, and/or mental status changes. If the pneumonia is severe, it can also cause respiratory distress, confusion and/or obtundation. A physician usually diagnoses pneumonia on the basis of a chest x-ray, arterial blood gas (ABG), and other lab tests. The treatment for pneumonia almost always includes antibiotics.

There are a variety of classification schemes that have been used to categorize the various types of pneumonia, most of which are based on the clinical circumstances in which the pneumonia occurs. For instance, pneumonia is sometimes classified according to where it occurs, for example, community acquired pneumonia (CAP) or hospital-acquired pneumonia (HAP). Ventilator-associated pneumonia (VAP) is a subtype of HAP in this classification scheme. Pneumonia can also be classified by the anatomic location in which it occurs, for example, lobar versus bronchial. Classification of pneumonia according the mechanism of acquisition

Table 5–2. Weakened Pulmonary Defenses: Risk Factors for Pneumonia

Impaired System	Contributing Factors
Weakened anatomic defenses	endotracheal intubation, tracheostomy
Diminished protective reflexes	stroke, brain injury, seizure, alcohol and/or drug intoxication, anesthesia
Reduced cough effectiveness	tetraplegia, neuromuscular disease, COPD, airway obstruction
Weakened mucocillary clearance	smoking, viral infection, COPD, bronchiectasis, excessive mucous (e.g., cystic fibrosis), inherited ciliary disorders, airway obstruction (e.g., endotracheostomy tube or tumor), dehydration
Weakened immunologic defenses	HIV, transplant, immunosuppressive therapy, alcoholism, malnutrition, diabetes

is more familiar to the speech pathologist, for example, aspiration pneumonia versus hematogenous pneumonia versus pneumonia that occurs due to inhalation of toxic substances.

Types of Aspiration and Associated Pulmonary Sequelae

Aspiration is the entry of food or any type of liquid (including saliva or gastric contents) below the level of the vocal folds into the lower respiratory tract. Aspiration pneumonia may or may not occur following an aspiration event. There are additional factors to consider with respect to assessing one's risk for aspiration pneumonia. These include the integrity of one's pulmonary defenses, the volume and pH of the bolus aspirated and the presence/absence of pathogens. Common pathogens include bacteria, viruses, and fungi. Pathogens can also include toxic or noxious chemicals. Different pulmonary syndromes can occur following aspiration, depending on the amount, frequency, and content of the aspirated substance (Marik, 2001). It is important to distinguish among a few types of aspiration related pulmonary sequelae, including distinguishing aspiration pneumonia from aspiration pneumonitis, asphyxiation due to a "cafe coronary syndrome," lung disease due to chronic microaspiration, and the nosocomial ventilator-associated pneumonia (VAP).

Aspiration pneumonia is "an infectious process caused by the inhalation of oropharyngeal secretions that are colonized by pathogenic bacteria" (Marik, 2001). Conversely, aspiration pneumonitis, also known as "Mendelson syndrome," is a chemical injury to the lung parenchyma that occurs due to aspiration of sterile gastric contents (Marik, 2001). The pathophysiology and clinical signs/symptoms differ between aspiration pneumonia and aspiration pneumonitis. Aspiration pneumonitis tends to occur during a markedly reduced level of consciousness, for example, during anesthesia, coma, drug overdose, or seizure (Marik, 2001). It results in acute lung injury and/or chemical burns to lung parenchyma from gastric and particulate matter that has high acidity levels (i.e., pH <2.5). The severity of the injury is more profound as pH decreases and volume of aspirate increases. Aspiration of particulate food matter from the stomach can result in severe lung damage. In these cases, respiratory distress typically occurs within 2 to 5 hours following the aspiration event. In contrast, aspiration pneumonia is more frequently associated with dysphagia, gastroesophageal reflux, and/or aspiration of bacteria-laden secretions (Marik, 2001). It is characterized by a pulmonary inflammatory response to bacteria and bacteria products. Aspiration of food is more likely to be associated with pneumonia than aspiration of liquid (Langmore et al., 1998). Additionally, there is a correlation between the volume of aspirate and the development of aspiration pneumonia (Marik, 2001).

One primary source of bacteria that can contribute to aspiration pneumonia is that contained in the oral cavity. Institutionalized patients are at greater risk of developing colonization of dental plaque with respiratory pathogens than are community dwelling outpatients (Scannapieco, 2006). In fact, oropharyngeal flora and microbes can change within 48 hours of admission to an intensive care unit (Halm & Armola, 2009). Possible contributing factors include use of antibiotics and xerostomia. Antibiotics can reduce other commensal flora, or nonpathogenic bacteria, that compete with pathogens for colonization. Xerostomia can inhibit mucocillary function and reduce the protective aspects of saliva. In nursing homes and hospitals, oral care is sometimes neglected for patients who are unable to complete this task independently. Studies have revealed that in nursing homes mechanical cleaning with a toothbrush of the teeth or dentures, tongue, roof of mouth, and other oral structures has resulted in a reduction of bacteria in the oral cavity. Consequently, significantly fewer people with pneumonia and death due to aspiration pneumonia have been reported (Ishikawa, Yoneyama, Hirota, Miyake, & Miyatake, 2008; Yoneyama et al., 2002). Despite this knowledge, nursing home staffs are sometimes reluctant to perform oral care for people that are known to aspirate for fear of aspiration during oral care. In these cases, the speech pathologist can assist with teaching aspiration precautions that can be used during oral care, for example, upright position with neck slightly flexed (chin down), use of suction simultaneous with oral care, or a toothbrush attached to suction.

The phrase "cafe coronary," coined by Haugen in 1963, refers to sudden death that occurs due to occlusion of the airway by food. Based on medical and autopsy records of individuals that have died of asphyxiation from food blocking the airway, a pattern of risk factors for cafe coronary has emerged. Autopsy records of those who have died of cafe coronary revealed high percentages of people with neurologic and/or psychiatric disorders and the elderly (Berzlanovich, Fazeny-Dorner, Waldhoer, Fasching, & Keil, 2005; Wick, Gilbert, & Byard, 2006). Berzlanovich et al. (2005) reported that nursing

home residents represented the highest number of food asphyxiation deaths in the Adelaide, Australia community over a 10-year period. Additional risk factors include absent or sparse dentition, alcohol intoxication, medications (sedative, psychotropic and/or anticholinergic, and dopaminergic medications), xerostomia, and the type of food being ingested (Berzlanovich et al., 2005; Wick et al., 2006). The most common type of food resulting in asphyxiation was large chunks of solid foods, such as mixed solid foods and/or large single chunks of meat (Berzlanovich et al., 2005). However, in the elderly population, semisolid (i.e., pureed) foods have resulted in a large number of asphyxiation deaths as well (Wick et al., 2006). Risk factors for asphyxiation from food, specific to dysphagia signs and symptoms, were studied in a population of adults with intellectual disabilities and dysphagia, for example, a subgroup with cerebral palsy and those with Down syndrome (Samuels & Chadwick, 2006). In this study asphyxiation risk was determined by medical record documentation indicating significant instances of choking episodes. The following factors were determined to be predictive of asphyxiation risk: maladaptive eating behaviors of "cramming" and eating at a rapid speed, and the physiological observation of premature spillage of the bolus into the pharynx, that is, prior to initiation of the swallow (Samuels & Chadwick, 2006).

Silent microaspiration can occur in up to 50% of the normal population during sleep (Gleeson, Eggli, & Maxwell, 1997). However, recent studies suggest a possible link between microaspiration of gastric reflux and a variety of lung diseases, including idiopathic pulmonary fibrosis (IPF) (Lee et al., 2010). IPF is characterized by chronic fibrosis of the lungs. There is no cure and median survival is 2 to 3 years. This hypothesis that chronic microaspiration of reflux might be associated with IPF is based, in part, on research showing a strong association between gastroesophageal reflux disease (GERD) and IPF, and animal research showing a relationship between chronic aspiration and pulmonary fibrosis (Lee et al., 2010). However, most people with GERD do not present with IPF. Therefore, further research is needed to confirm or refute the link between microaspiration of reflux and lung diseases, such as IPF.

VAP, the form of aspiration pneumonia that frequently occurs in people that are intubated for ventilator support, is the second most common infection in critically ill patients. Depending on other underlying diagnoses, VAP contributes significantly to mortality (Palmer, 2009). There several reasons for the high risk of aspiration pneumonia in this population. Oropharyngeal flora and microbes can change within 48 hours of admission to an intensive care unit (Halm & Armola, 2009). Ventilator tubing, inserted intraorally and between the vocal folds and down into the airway, blocks vocal fold closure, a key pulmonary defense. Despite efforts to block aspiration with a fully inflated cuff, colonized secretions pool above the cuff and frequently leak to the lower airway via creases and/or other leaks in the seal of the cuff (Palmer, 2009). In addition, the process of intubation and the cuff itself often result in injury to laryngeal and tracheal tissues. Impaired mucociliary clearance, supine positioning, and sedation are all contributing factors. Completing oral care is often challenging and the risk for reflux can be higher in critically ill patients (Palmer, 2009). All of these factors combine to dramatically increase the risk for aspiration pneumonia. Efforts to prevent VAP include elevating the head of the bed, reflux prophylaxis, increasing periods of reduced sedation, clearing subglottic secretions, and weaning the patient from mechanical ventilation as soon as possible (Palmer, 2009).

RESPIRATORY ASSESSMENT FOR A SWALLOWING EVALUATION

Within the context of a swallowing evaluation, respiratory assessment begins with a medical records review. The clinician should make note of diagnoses and/or conditions that might affect the integrity of one's pulmonary defenses, as well as respiratory evaluation data collected by other professionals. Tables 5–2 and 5–3 present examples of conditions that can impair various aspects of an individual's pulmonary defenses. Documentation of respiratory related evaluation results from the covering physician, pulmonary medicine specialist, and/or respiratory

---

Table 5–3. Factors That Can Inhibit Mucocillary Clearance

- Smoking
- Infection (e.g. Influenza virus)
- Abnormal mucus (e.g. cystic fibrosis)
- Abnormal cilia (e.g. immotile cilia syndrome)
- Obstruction (e.g. endotracheostomy tube, tumor)
- Dehydration
- Xerostomia

therapists should be reviewed when available. This might include results of pulmonary function tests, arterial blood gases (ABGs), chest x-ray, and/or other imaging tests involving the thoracic region. Selected portions of a respiratory assessment are briefly summarized below.

Pulmonary function tests (PFTs) refer to a battery of tests that provide information on the functional status of the respiratory system. Spirometry is the most commonly employed procedure in the PFT battery. Using a spirometer, airflow is measured during a variety of breathing tasks, including how much and how fast air can be moved in and out of the lungs (Al-Ashkar, Mehra, & Mazzone, 2003). This information aids differential diagnosis, for example, distinguishing restrictive versus obstructive respiratory disorders, and screening for the possibility of airway obstruction. In the context of rehabilitation, PFTs are sometimes used to monitor progression of respiratory dysfunction, and/or to measure the effectiveness of treatment. In Figure 5–2, a volume-time graph demonstrates the various lung volumes and capacities. Normal values for PFTs can vary with certain variables, including age, gender and height. Therefore, the results of PFTs typically are reported in percents of that expected for a given individual. The most important measures for distinguishing restrictive versus obstructive versus normal patterns are forced vital capacity (FVC), forced expiratory volume in 1 second (FEV_1) and the FEV_1/FVC ratio. FVC is a measure of the volume of air that can be forcefully expired following a maximal inspiratory effort. FEV_1 is the amount of air exhaled during the first second of the FVC task. Then the FEV_1/FVC ratio is used to rule in or out an obstructive pattern (Al-Ashkar, et al., 2003). Distinguishing features between obstructive and restrictive patterns are illustrated in Table 5–4.

Spirometry data may be presented graphically in the form of a volume by time curve or a *flow-volume loop*, with volume on the x-axis and flow (liters/second) on the y-axis. Patterns may indicate specific diagnoses. For instance, a pattern associated with obstructive disorders, such as COPD, is characterized by a slower pattern of exhalation. Conversely, restrictive patterns typically reveal a reduction in overall volume. In Figure 5–6, flow-volume loops are demonstrated for normal versus obstructive and restrictive pulmonary conditions.

Patterns shown via the flow-volume loop may indicate the presence of an upper airway obstruction, including obstruction at the level of the vocal folds. Three characteristic flow-volume loop

Table 5–4. Obstructive or Restrictive Patterns		
Measure	*Obstructive pattern*	*Restrictive pattern*
FVC	Decreased or normal	Decrease
FEV_1	Decreased	Decreased or normal
FEV_1/FVC ratio	Decreased	Normal
Total Lung Capacity (TLC)	Normal or increased	Decreased

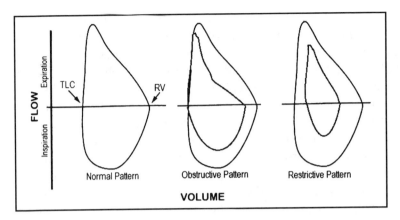

Figure 5–6. Flow-volume loop—Obstructive versus restrictive patterns. With obstructive lung diseases, such as COPD, a concave flow-volume loop pattern is typically seen, as it takes longer for the patient to exhale due to airflow obstruction. With restrictive breathing disorders, the total lung volume will be lower. This can occur due to weakened respiratory muscles, for example, cervical spinal cord injury, and/or conditions that reduce lung compliance, for example, pulmonary fibrosis.

patterns are well known (Figure 5-7). However, several studies have reported that visual inspection for patterns on flow-volume loops has demonstrated poor sensitivity for detection of upper airway obstruction (Modrykamien, Gudavalli, McCarthy, Liu, & Stoller, 2009). Additionally, abnormalities of the inspiratory loop can occur due to inadequate effort (Sterner, Morris, Sill, & Hayes, 2009). Therefore, clinicians should not solely rely on flow-loop information, especially if upper airway dysfunction is suspected. Despite this, the observation of abnormal patterns can indicate upper airway disease and should prompt further assessment.

Vincken et al. (1986) reported that abnormal flow-volume loops characterized by inspiratory and/or expiratory flow limitations and inspiratory or expiratory flow oscillations (saw tooth pattern) could distinguish patients with bulbar involvement in neuromuscular disease

with good sensitivity and specificity (Vincken, Dollfuss, & Cosio, 1986). However, in a study comparing pulmonologist determinations of vocal fold dysfunction from flow-volume loops and other selected spirometry values with an endoscopic assessment of vocal fold dysfunction, none of the spirometric measures were predictive of vocal fold dysfunction (Watson, King, Holley, Greenburg, & Mikita, 2009). Thus, although it is clear that bulbar dysfunction can affect flow-volume loop patterns, research is needed to further elucidate causes for specific patterns.

For patients with suspected weakness of the respiratory muscles, it is helpful to isolate impairments of respiratory muscle strength from conditions involving the lungs (Evans & Whitelaw, 2009). Clinical measures of maximal respiratory mouth pressures are noninvasive and can be obtained efficiently in clinic. Maximal respiratory mouth pressures are more

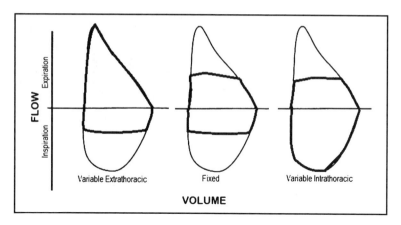

Figure 5–7. Flow-volume loops typical of various types of upper airway obstruction. A plateau associated with inspiration characterizes a variable extrathoracic upper airway obstruction (*left*). Potential causes for this type of obstruction are vocal fold paralysis or dysfunction. Flow plateaus during both inspiration and expiration characterize a fixed upper airway obstruction (above or within the thorax) (*center*). Potential causes for this type of obstruction include large fixed tumors in the airway or goiter. A flow plateau associated with expiration characterizes a variable intrathoracic upper airway obstruction (*right*). A potential cause for this type of obstruction is a tumor or tracheomalacia in the intrathoracic airway.

sensitive than PFTs to early changes in respiratory muscle strength in people with neuromuscular disease (Evans & Whitelaw, 2009). Maximum inspiratory pressure (MIP) is used to measure inspiratory muscle strength. Maximum expiratory pressure (MEP) measures expiratory muscle strength. Both measures require that the individual insert a flanged mouthpiece orally while occluding the nares with a nose clip. In cases of severe oral weakness, a mask can be used in lieu of the mouthpiece. The mouthpiece is connected to a manometer; a small leak in the mouthpiece prevents inadvertent measurement of pressures generated intraorally. To measure MIP, the individual begins inspiratory effort at residual lung volume against a blocked airway. To measure MEP, the individual begins expiratory effort at

total lung capacity (TLC), again against a blocked airway. High measures are reliable for excluding respiratory muscle weakness. Some controversy exists about whether lower numbers for some might result from inadequate effort. If invalid findings are suspected, maximal inspiratory sniff pressure can also measure inspiratory muscle strength. Even with the additional measures, the lower limits of normal in these measures are still vague (Evans & Whitelaw, 2009). Similar to PFTs, normal values for MIP and MEP must be adjusted for age and sex (Evans & Whitelaw, 2009).

PFTs and maximal respiratory mouth pressures depend on a maximal level of effort being put forth by the patient. In certain neurologic populations volitional initiation of effort is impaired. This is found in patients with severe primary progressive multiple sclerosis, severe brain injury with subcortical and/or brainstem involvement, and severe oral apraxia associated with left brain stroke. Therefore, it might be difficult to collect valid PFT and/or maximal respiratory mouth pressures in patients with these conditions.

In assessing respiratory function it is important to clarify hypoxia-related terminology (Pierson, 2000). Hypoxemia refers to a reduced PaO_2 (partial pressure of oxygen in arterial blood). Hypoxia typically refers to a deficiency in the amount of oxygen supply to the tissues of the body (short of anoxia). Anoxia refers to an absence or near complete absence of oxygen supply to the tissues of the body. It is possible to have hypoxia without hypoxemia, for example, anemic hypoxia. However, hypoxemia is the most common cause of hypoxia.

Oxygen saturation (SaO_2) and respiratory rate are easy to monitor at bedside and can be helpful in determining a patient's tolerance of the swallowing evaluation, as well as monitoring overall breathing adequacy. In the intensive care unit, these data are continuously displayed for each patient. Pulse oximeters are a non-invasive way to measure oxyhemoglobin saturation (SaO_2), that is, how much oxygen is bound to hemoglobin (Figure 5–8). Normal SaO_2 range is from 90 to 100 mm Hg. With respect to monitoring SaO_2 during evaluation of swallowing, it is important to acknowledge that SaO_2 does not accurately predict aspiration (Wang, Chang, Chen, & Hsiao, 2005).

Normal respiratory rate for adults is 12 to 20 breaths per minute. Respiratory rate prior to and following swallowing can provide some additional information regarding the patient's coordination of

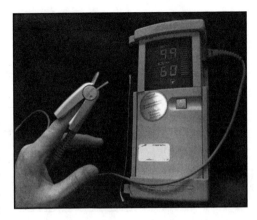

Figure 5–8. Pulse oximeter. The pulse oximeter measures oxygen saturation. Although it can provide useful information in determining a patient's breathing status, it does not detect aspiration during the swallow examination.

breathing and swallowing. For instance, if respiratory rate increases from 20 to 30 breaths per minute after a single swallow, this might indicate inefficiency in breathing swallowing coordination and that the period of apnea needed to swallow may be competing with respiratory needs.

Arterial blood gas (ABG) is a blood test frequently ordered to aid respiratory assessment. The results are presented as numbers in the following order: pH, PCO_2, HCO_3, PO_2. Table 5–5 presents normal ranges. Measures of blood pH (potential of hydrogen ion concentration) indicate overall acidity versus basicity level of the blood. PCO_2 is the partial pressure carbon dioxide. This can also be monitored noninvasively via nasal canula measures of end-tidal CO_2. HCO_3 is a measure of bicarbonate ions in the blood, which indicates metabolic acidity or basicity. PO_2 is partial pressure oxygen in the blood (normal = 90–100 mm Hg).

Physicians use ABG data to aid differential diagnosis of underlying respiratory disorders and causes for hypoxemia. Using the alveolar gas equation as explained in Table 5–6, physicians can quickly calculate the alveolar-arterial oxygen difference. This in turn aids determination of an underlying cause for hypoxemia. Some possible causes for hypoxemia, each characterized in part by variable patterns in the Alveolar-arterial (A-a) oxygen difference, are listed as follows: (1) Reduced partial pressure of inspired oxygen (P_IO_2), for example, breathing at a very high altitude with inadequate oxygen; (2) Hypoventilation, for example, inability to ventilate adequately due to restrictive respiratory dysfunction; (3) Ventilation/blood perfusion (V/Q) mismatch: typically a lower V/Q contributes to hypoxemia, for example, reduced gas exchange due to COPD or pulmonary fibrosis; and (4) Shunt (V/Q = 0, that is, no gas is being exchanged), for example, collapsed or fluid filled alveoli such as might occur with pneumonia and/or atelectasis. In cases where shunt is the underlying cause of hypoxemia, breathing additional oxygen does not help.

When pneumonia is suspected, a chest x-ray typically is ordered for further assessment. The site of pneumonia involvement on a chest x-ray can vary depending on the position of the person during

Table 5–5. Arterial Blood Gas (ABG) — Normal Values		
pH	*PCO_2 (Carbon Dioxide)*	*HCO_3 (Bicarbonate)*
• WNL: 7.4± .03 units	• WNL: 40± 3 mm Hg	• WNL: 24± 2 mEq/L
• Higher = alkalotic	• >45 = respiratory acidosis = hypoventilation	• Higher = metabolic alkalosis
• Lower = acidotic	• <35 = respiratory alkalosis = hyperventilation	• Lower = metabolic acidosis

Table 5–6. Alveolar Gas Equation	
$$P_AO_2 = P_IO_2 - \frac{P_aCO_2}{R}$$ Once P_AO_2 is estimated using the alveolar gas equation, the A-a oxygen difference is calculated, i.e., $P_AO_2 - P_IO_2$	P_AO_2: Partial pressure alveolar O_2 P_IO_2: Partial pressure inspired O_2 (varies depending on altitude) P_aCO_2: Arterial partial pressure CO_2 R = respiratory quotient (usually assumed to be 0.8); technically refers to the ratio of CO_2 produced to O_2 consumed per unit time in the body under stable conditions. A = alveolar a = arterial

aspiration (Marik, 2001). For patients who aspirate while in a recumbent position, the posterior portions of the upper lobes tend to infiltrate, whereas those that aspirate in upright positions tend to have segments of the lower lobes more affected. Regardless of the site of involvement, medical treatment is needed to prevent further damage.

Speech Pathology Respiratory Exam

Based on observations and an interview with the patient, the clinician concerned with swallowing should note whether the patient is reporting or demonstrating any possible signs or symptoms of hypoventilation and/or hypoxia (Table 5–7).

Selection of respiratory evaluation components will depend in part on what has already been assessed by other professionals on the multidisciplinary team. For instance, if the respiratory therapist recently assessed cough strength for a particular patient, it is not necessary to repeat this. In this instance, the clinician will be most efficient by making use of available multidisciplinary data. In addition, completion of the respiratory exam will in part depend on which components the examiner is competent to complete. When the clinician concerned with swallowing cannot complete needed portions of the exam, in some cases it might be appropriate to refer the evaluation to the team. For instance, if pulmonary function tests have not been collected for a patient with motor neuron disease, the these clinician could collect these data if they have been trained in spirometry or simply measure slow vital capacity (VC). Slow

Table 5–7. Possible Indications of Inadequate Ventilation and/or Hypoxia

Behavioral Observations	Physical Signs	Patient complaints*
• Drowsiness*	• Weak cough	• Dyspnea (i.e., shortness of breath) at rest or with talking and/or with exertion (e.g., walking)
• Lethargy*	• Tachypnea (i.e., rapid breathing rate)	
• Confusion		• Orthopnea (i.e., dyspnea) when lying flat
• Restlessness	• Stridor (i.e., hearing phonation on inhalation)	
• Agitation	• Paradoxic breathing patterns	• Fatigue
• Memory or attention impairments*	• Difficulty clearing secretions*	• Headache pain
	• Tachycardia (i.e., rapid heartbeat)	• Hallucinations
	• Tremor*	• Difficulty sleeping
	• Diaphoresis* (i.e., excessive sweating)	• Depression
		• Palpitations

*May also be a patient complaint.
Source: From Leigh et al., 2003; Pierson, 2000.

VC can be measured easily with a hand-held respirometer and requires little training (Daykin, Nunn, & Wright, 1978). If unable to collect these data, the clinician can recommend that another competent professional on the team assess the patient's current pulmonary status.

Examination of respiratory support typically includes VC in upright and supine positions, and measures of peak expiratory cough flow (PECF). Measures of sustained phonation, spoken syllables per breath and perceptual voice quality data provide information on respiratory support for speech combined with voice function. PECF can be measured with a peak expiratory flow meter with an air cushion face mask (Figure 5–9) (Boitano, 2006). Although norms are not yet available for PECF, >160 L per min has been reported to be required for adequate secretion clearance for purposes of extubation (Bach & Saporito, 1996), and persons with <270 L per min are considered

to be at risk for respiratory complications (Bach, Ishikawa, & Kim, 1997). As indicated above, it is important to acknowledge that reflexive cough strength frequently is different from volitional cough strength in people with neuromuscular disease.

SUMMARY

Consideration of respiratory function, pulmonary defenses and background medical information is vital to the evaluation and treatment of swallowing. This information will aid the clinical assessment of an individual's overall risk for aspiration. An individual's swallowing function must be considered within the context of the individual's overall risk for aspiration pneumonia. Considering the patient's risk for pneumonia and/or other pulmonary sequelae will also facilitate appropriate treatment planning.

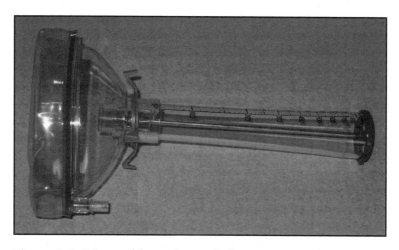

Figure 5–9. Disposable peak-cough-flow meter with face-mask attached. Use of a disposable peak-cough-flow meter is a quick, and inexpensive, way to measure peak expiratory cough flow (PECF). For patients with poor lip seal, a mask can be attached to aid measurement.

REFERENCES

Al-Ashkar, F., Mehra, R., & Mazzone, P. J. (2003). Interpreting pulmonary function tests: recognize the pattern, and the diagnosis will follow. *Cleveland Clinic Journal of Medicine, 70*(10), 866, 868, 871-873, 877-881.

Bach, J. R., Ishikawa, Y., & Kim, H. (1997). Prevention of pulmonary morbidity for patients with Duchenne muscular dystrophy. *Chest, 112*(4), 1024-1028.

Bach, J. R., & Saporito, L. R. (1996). Criteria for extubation and tracheostomy tube removal for patients with ventilatory failure: A different approach to weaning. *Chest, 110*(6), 1566-1571.

Bals, R., Weiner, D. J., & Wilson, J. M. (1999). The innate immune system in cystic fibrosis lung disease. *Journal of Clinical Investigation, 103*(3), 303-307.

Baydur, A., Adkins, R. H., & Milic-Emili, J. (2001). Lung mechanics in individuals with spinal cord injury: Effects of injury level and posture. *Journal of Applied Physiology, 90*(2), 405-411.

Berzlanovich, A. M., Fazeny-Dorner, B., Waldhoer, T., Fasching, P., & Keil, W. (2005). Foreign body asphyxia: A preventable cause of death in the elderly. *American Journal of Preventive Medicine, 28*(1), 65-69.

Boden, K., Cedborg, A. I., Eriksson, L. I., Hedstrom, H. W., Kuylenstierna, R., Sundman, E., & Ekberg, O. (2009). Swallowing and respiratory pattern in young healthy individuals recorded with high temporal resolution. *Neurogastroenterology and Motility, 21*(11), e1163-e1101.

Boitano, L. J. (2006). Management of airway clearance in neuromuscular disease. *Respiratory Care, 51*(8), 913-924.

Charbonneau, I., Lund, J. P., & McFarland, D. H. (2005). Persistence of respiratory-swallowing coordination after laryngectomy. *Journal of Speech, Language, and Hearing Research, 48*(1), 34-44.

Daykin, A. P., Nunn, G. F., & Wright, B. M. (1978). The measurement of vital capacity and minute volume with the Wright respirometer. *British Journal of Disorders of the Chest, 22*, 333-335.

Dozier, T. S., Brodsky, M. B., Michel, Y., Walters, B. C., Jr., & Martin-Harris, B. (2006). Coordination of swallowing and respiration in normal sequential cup swallows. *Laryngoscope, 116*(8), 1489-1493.

Evans, J. A., & Whitelaw, W. A. (2009). The assessment of maximal respiratory mouth pressures in adults. *Respiratory Care, 54*(10), 1348-1359.

Finder, J. D. (2010). Airway clearance modalities in neuromuscular disease. *Pediatric Respiratory Review, 11*(1), 31-34.

Gleeson, K., Eggli, D. F., & Maxwell, S. L. (1997). Quantitative aspiration during sleep in normal subjects. *Chest, 111*(5), 1266-1272.

Gross, R. D. (2009). Subglottic air pressure and swallowing. *Perspectives on Swallowing and Swallowing Disorders (Dysphagia), 18*, 13-18.

Hadjikoutis, S., Pickersgill, T. P., Dawson, K., & Wiles, C. M. (2000). Abnormal patterns of breathing during swallowing in neurological disorders. *Brain, 123*(Pt. 9), 1863-1873.

Halm, M. A., & Armola, R. (2009). Effect of oral care on bacterial colonization and ventilator-associated pneumonia. *American Journal of Critical Care, 18*(3), 275-278.

Happel, K. I., Bagby, G. J., & Nelson, S. (2004). Host defense and bacterial pneumonia. *Seminars Respiratory Critical Care Medicine, 25*(1), 43-52.

Hillel, A. D. (2001). The study of laryngeal muscle activity in normal human subjects and in patients with laryngeal dystonia using multiple fine-wire electromyography. *Laryngoscope, 111*(4 Pt. 2, Suppl. 97), 1-47.

Hiss, S. G., Strauss, M., Treole, K., Stuart, A., & Boutilier, S. (2003). Swallowing apnea as a function of airway closure. *Dysphagia, 18*(4), 293-300.

Ishikawa, A., Yoneyama, T., Hirota, K., Miyake, Y., & Miyatake, K. (2008). Professional oral health care reduces the number of oropharyngeal bacteria. *Journal of Dental Research, 87*(6), 594–598.

Langmore, S. E., Terpenning, M. S., Schork, A., Yinmiao, C., Murray, J. T., Lopatin, D., & Loesche, W. J. (1998). Predictors of aspiration pneumonia: How important is dysphagia? *Dysphagia, 13*, 69–81.

Lasserson, D., Mills, K., Arunachalam, R., Polkey, M., Moxham, J., & Kalra, L. (2006). Differences in motor activation of voluntary and reflex cough in humans. *Thorax, 61*(8), 699–705.

Lee, J. S., Collard, H. R., Raghu, G., Sweet, M. P., Hays, S. R., Campos, G. M., . . . King, T. E. Jr. (2010). Does chronic microaspiration cause idiopathic pulmonary fibrosis? *American Journal of Medicine, 123*(4), 304–311.

Leigh, P. N., Abrahams, S., Al-Chalabi, A., Ampong, M. A., Goldstein, L. H., Johnson, J., . . . Willey, E..(2003). The management of motor neurone disease. *Journal of Neurology and Neurosurgery Psychiatry, 74* (Suppl. 4), iv32–iv47.

Marik, P. E. (2001). Aspiration pneumonitis and aspiration pneumonia. *New England Journal of Medicine, 344*(9), 665–671.

Martin, B. J., Logemann, J. A., Shaker, R., & Dodds, W. J. (1994). Coordination between respiration and swallowing: Respiratory phase relationships and temporal integration. *Journal of Applied Physiology, 76*(2), 714–723.

Martin-Harris, B. (2008). Clinical implications of respiratory-swallowing interactions. *Current Opinions in Otolaryngology and Head and Neck Surgery, 16*(3), 194–199.

Martin-Harris, B., Brodsky, M. B., Michel, Y., Ford, C. L., Walters, B., & Heffner, J. (2005). Breathing and swallowing dynamics across the adult lifespan. *Archives of Otolaryngology-Head and Neck Surgery, 131*(9), 762–770.

Martin-Harris, B., Brodsky, M. B., Price, C. C., Michel, Y., & Walters, B. (2003). Temporal coordination of pharyngeal and laryngeal dynamics with breathing during swallowing: single liquid swallows. *Journal of Applied Physiology, 94*(5), 1735–1743.

Matsuo, K., & Palmer, J. B. (2009). Coordination of mastication, swallowing and breathing. *Japanese Dental Science Review, 45*(1), 31–40.

Modrykamien, A. M., Gudavalli, R., McCarthy, K., Liu, X., & Stoller, J. K. (2009). Detection of upper airway obstruction with spirometry results and the flow-volume loop: A comparison of quantitative and visual inspection criteria. *Respiratory Care, 54*(4), 474–479.

Nishino, T., & Hiraga, K. (1991). Coordination of swallowing and respiration in unconscious subjects. *Journal of Applied Physiology, 70*(3), 988–993.

Palmer, L. B. (2009). Ventilator-associated infection. *Current Opinion in Pulmonary Medicine, 15*(3), 230–235.

Pierson, D. J. (1992). Respiratory failure: Introduction and Overview. In D. J. Pierson & R. M. Kacmarek (Eds.), *Foundations of respiratory care* (pp. 295–302). New York, NY: Churchill Livingstone.

Pierson, D. J. (2000). Pathophysiology and clinical effects of chronic hypoxia. *Respiratory Care, 45*(1), 39–51; discussion 51–33.

Poletto, C. J., Verdun, L. P., Strominger, R., & Ludlow, C. L. (2004). Correspondence between laryngeal vocal fold movement and muscle activity during speech and nonspeech gestures. *Journal of Applied Physiology, 97*(3), 858–866.

Preiksaitis, H. G., Mayrand, S., Robins, K., & Diamant, N. E. (1992). Coordination of respiration and swallowing: Effect of bolus volume in normal adults. *American Journal of Physiology, 263*(3 Pt. 2), R624–R630.

Qureshi, A. (2009). Diaphragm paralysis. *Seminars in Respiratory Critical Care Medicine, 30*(3), 315–320.

Samuels, R., & Chadwick, D. D. (2006). Predictors of asphyxiation risk in adults with intellectual disabilities and dysphagia. *Journal of Intellectual Disability Research, 50* (Pt. 5), 362–370.

Scannapieco, F. A. (2006). Pneumonia in nonambulatory patients. The role of oral bacteria and oral hygiene. *Journal of the American Dental Association*, *137*(Supplement), 21S–25S.

Selley, W. G., Flack, F. C., Ellis, R. E., & Brooks, W. A. (1989). Respiratory patterns associated with swallowing: Part 1. The normal adult pattern and changes with age. *Age and Ageing*, *18*(3), 168–172.

Smith-Hammond, C. (2008). Cough and aspiration of food and liquids due to oral pharyngeal dysphagia. *Lung*, *186*(Suppl. 1), S35–S40.

Smith-Hammond, C., Goldstein, L. B., Horner, R. D., Ying, J., Gray, L., Gonzalez-Rothi, L., & Bolser, D. C. (2009). Predicting aspiration in patients with ischemic stroke: Comparison of clinical signs and aerodynamic measures of voluntary cough. *Chest*, *135*(3), 769–777.

Stephens, R. E., Addington, W. R., & Widdicombe, J. G. (2003). Effect of acute unilateral middle cerebral artery infarcts on voluntary cough and the laryngeal cough reflex. *American Journal of Physical Medicine and Rehabilitation*, *82*(5), 379–383.

Sterner, J. B., Morris, M. J., Sill, J. M., & Hayes, J. A. (2009). Inspiratory flow-volume curve evaluation for detecting upper airway disease. *Respiratory Care*, *54*(4), 461–466.

Terzi, N., Orlikowski, D., Aegerter, P., Lejaille, M., Ruquet, M., Zalcman, G., . . . Lofaso, F. (2007). Breathing-swallowing interaction in neuromuscular patients: A physiological evaluation. *American Journal of Respiratory and Critical Care Medicine*, *175*(3), 269–276.

Vincken, W., Dollfuss, R. E., & Cosio, M. G. (1986). Upper airway dysfunction detected by respiratory flow oscillations. *European Journal of Respiratory Diseases*, *68*(1), 50–57.

von Leden, H., & Isshiki, N. (1965). An analysis of cough at the level of the larynx. *Archives of Otolaryngology*, *81*, 616–625.

Wang, T. G., Chang, Y. C., Chen, S. Y., & Hsiao, T. Y. (2005). Pulse oximetry does not reliably detect aspiration on videofluoroscopic swallowing study. *Archives of Physical Medicine and Rehabilitation*, *86*(4), 730–734.

Watson, M. A., King, C. S., Holley, A. B., Greenburg, D. L., & Mikita, J. A. (2009). Clinical and lung-function variables associated with vocal cord dysfunction. *Respiratory Care*, *54*(4), 467–473.

Wick, R., Gilbert, J. D., & Byard, R. W. (2006). Cafe coronary syndrome-fatal choking on food: An autopsy approach. *Journal of Clinical Forensic Medicine*, *13*(3), 135–138.

Yoneyama, T., Yoshida, M., Ohrui, T., Mukaiyama, H., Okamoto, H., Hoshiba, K., . . . Sasaki, H. (2002). Oral care reduces pneumonia in older patients in nursing homes. *Journal of the American Geriatrics Society*, *50*(3), 430–433.

6 The Use of Instrumental Examinations in Neuromuscular Diseases

There are many good reviews in the literature of videofluoroscopic (VFS) and fiberoptic examinations for dysphagia that outline procedures and protocols (Aviv & Murry, 2005, Langmore, Schatz, & Olson, 1988, Leonard & Kendall, 2007, Murray, 1999). In particular, the chapters on videofluoroscopy and videoendoscopy in the companion text in this series, *Dysphagia in Movement Disorders*, are recommended (Rosenbek & Jones, 2009). This chapter provides guidance in the general application of these examinations for patients with neuromuscular diseases. Because most of these diseases are degenerative in nature, clinicians are faced with symptoms that develop and progress at varying rates over time. Among the questions that arise regarding the use of instrumental examinations for patients with neuromuscular diseases are: What are the indicators for performing an instrumental examination? When an examination is warranted, how often should it be repeated? How should findings be interpreted in light of constantly changing symptoms?

In Chapter 4 (Clinical Swallowing Examination), the point was made that the clinical assessment provides clues relative to the underlying neuromuscular diagnosis whereas instrumental examinations are more limited in this regard. The strengths of instrumental examinations are the visualization of structures and the recordings of dynamic movements that allow for analysis of the biomechanics of swallowing. Certainly, there are correlations between biomechanics and underlying neuromuscular impairments, however, an appreciation for the presence of abnormalities in muscle tone, force, and range of movement requires the integration of data obtained during the clinical examination. Conversely, instrumental examinations, particularly those utilizing dynamic radiographic imaging, can: (1) assess structures that cannot be visualized on the clinical examination, for example, the upper esophageal sphincter and esophagus; (2) visualize bolus movement through the oral, pharyngeal and esophageal cavities; (3) visually detect misdirection of the bolus, particularly airway penetration and aspiration; and (4) assess timing of movement and the interactions between structures. If not for the expense, logistical issues, accessibility, and minor risks associated with x-ray exposure, patients could undergo VFS and clinical examinations routinely and the clinician would be consistently provided with data sufficient to describe both the dynamics of swallowing and the neuromuscular state at any given moment in time. Unfortunately, the factors that limit use of VFS, and to a lesser extent endoscopy, exist and influence clinical practice.

INDICATORS FOR PERFORMING AN INSTRUMENTAL EXAMINATION

The American Speech-Language-Hearing Association (ASHA) has published guidelines describing the indicators for conducting an instrumental examination. Inherent in these guidelines is the supposition that a clinical examination was administered as the first step in the assessment process. In fact, it is the findings from the clinical examination that should guide the process of the instrumental examination. ASHA's six indicators address the following issues: (1) a patient's signs and symptoms are inconsistent with findings on the clinical examination; (2) confirmation is needed for a suspected medical diagnosis and/or to assist in the determination of a differential medical diagnosis; (3) confirmation and/or differential diagnosis of the dysphagia is needed; (4) there is a question regarding the relative contribution of oropharyngeal dysphagia to a nutritional or pulmonary compromise; (5) safety and efficiency of swallowing remains a concern; and (6) swallowing rehabilitation is indicated and specific information is needed to guide intervention.

With the population of patients having neuromuscular diseases, this is particularly important to utilize reliable indicators to guide decisions regarding the use of instrumental examinations. Most of these clients will require a series of clinical examinations occurring throughout the course of their disease and clinicians must be judicious regarding the timing of instrumental examinations and base decisions on their finding from the clinical assessment.

The indicators listed in Table 6–1 are used to help guide our recommendations for an instrumental examination. As laryngeal endoscopy often is included as part of our clinical examinations, the following indicators listed apply primarily to the use of VFS studies.

In ASHA's document on "Clinical Indicators for Instrumental Assessment of Dysphagia" there are published stipulations regarding when instrumental examinations are not indicated. For example, one would not conduct an instrumental examination when clinical findings fail to identify dysphagia or the findings suggest: (a) the patient is too medically unstable to tolerate a procedure, (b) the patient is unable to cooperate or participate in an instrumental examination, or (c) in the clinician's judgment, the instrumental examination would not change the clinical management of the patient.

IMPORTANT DATA FROM THE INSTRUMENTAL EXAMINATION

At initial assessment, it is not so much a question of whether or not to perform an instrumental examination, but rather what questions need to be answered using data that are not accessible on clinical examination. In this way the instrumental examination can be tailored to answer specific questions that might relate to particular aspects of structural integrity, functional efficiency, and/or the effectiveness of compensatory postures and behaviors.

Although both VFS and endoscopic examinations provide valuable data, they are used to answer different questions.

Table 6–1. Indicators and Examples for Performing VFS Exams	
INDICATORS	**EXAMPLE**
There are inconsistencies between the patient's complaints and the findings of a clinical examination	Patient with a medical diagnosis of amyotrophic lateral sclerosis complains of difficulty with solids but not liquids; clinical exam shows neuromuscular weakness and incoordination consistent with medical diagnosis, but no explanation for dysphagia for solids
There are inconsistencies between findings documented on a clinical examination and established medical diagnosis	Medical diagnosis of repeat episodes of aspiration pneumonia in a patient with multiple sclerosis, but clinical exam shows no evidence of structural or functional impairment in oropharyngeal swallowing
Information is needed to confirm a medical diagnosis or provide data that are needed to formulate a medical diagnosis	Medical report states "probable impairment of upper esophageal sphincter opening due to known cervical osteophytes" for a patient in recovery phase of Guillain-Barré syndrome
There is need to either confirm or establish a differential diagnosis of dysphagia	Clinical inspection demonstrates velar weakness consistent with a diagnosed neuromuscular disease (e.g., myasthenia gravis), and patient complains of intermittent nasal-pharyngeal regurgitation
There is a need to determine the extent to which the presence of an oropharyngeal dysphagia is negatively impacting the health and welfare of the patient, particularly with regard to nutrition/hydration and pulmonary health	A patient with slowly progressive neuromuscular disease (e.g., autosomal dominant form of oculopharyngeal muscular dystrophy), has not had a bout of pneumonia, but reportedly has had an exacerbation of preexisting asthmatic complaints since the onset of swallowing difficulties
There is a need to determine the effectiveness and efficiency of the patient's oropharyngeal swallowing	In a patient with stable neuromuscular disease (e.g., myotonic muscular dystrophy), there has been reports of restricted diet and slow weight loss
Information regarding the effectiveness of postural adjustments, maneuvers, bolus modifications and/or other adjustments on improving the effectiveness and efficiency of swallowing	Patient with severe physical impairment due to long-standing neuromuscular disease (e.g., relapsing-remitting multiple sclerosis), needs demonstration of effective modifications of diet texture and the institution of maneuvers to improve swallowing efficiency
Data are required beyond the clinical examination to make recommendations regarding the appropriate mode(s) of nutritional management	Patient with a diagnosis of progressive bulbar palsy and the recent placement of a PEG tube seeks advice regarding the resumption of partial oral intake of food for pleasure

VFS provides important data in both the assessment process and potential treatment of patients with neuromuscular disease by allowing the visualization and recorded documentation of bolus movement through the entire oral-pharyngeal-esophageal deglutitory tract. To provide some degree of objectivity to the VFS, we recommend that clinicians employ the Penetration-Aspiration Scale (PAS) (Rosenbek, Robbins, Roecker, Coyle, & Wood, 1996).

Endoscopy documents only a portion of the swallowing mechanism, namely the inferior pharyngeal region and airway. Additionally, endoscopy does not allow for visualization of the bolus and structures at the height of the pharyngeal stage of swallowing, as there is a "whiteout" phenomenon that occurs to obscure the view.

The most common questions that arise following a clinical examination for patients with neuromuscular impairments that may be answered by an instrumental examination include the following: Do observable swallowing functions correspond to the patient's symptoms and the clinical examination? Are the biomechanics of swallowing consistent with the medical, neurologic diagnosis? Are recommended modifications of parameters such as diet and posture effective in producing more efficient and safer swallows? Are there any previously unidentified factors that might influence the patient's ability to effectively swallow?

The efficacy for the use of VFS to document a baseline of function in the early stages of most neuromuscular diseases is debatable. In those progressive neuromuscular disorders where the development of swallowing problems is very insidious, there may be few data obtained that could not have been charted by a careful clinical examination. In our own clinical practice, VFS documentation is not routinely obtained, as most pertinent baseline data is recorded from the clinical examination. However, instances exist when objective, reproducible data are very useful for later comparison. Clinical judgment should guide decisions regarding the use of instrumental examinations and the particular methodology employed. As the disease progresses, patients' specific symptoms will dictate whether or not VFS or endoscopy will provide useful information that will assist in applying appropriate interventions and recommendations.

REFERENCES

Aviv, J. E., & Murry, T. (2005). *FEEST: Flexible endoscopic evaluation of swallowing with sensory testing*. San Diego, CA: Plural.

Langmore, S. E., Schatz, K., & Olson, N. (1988). Fiberscopic endoscopic evaluation of swallowing safety. *Dysphagia, 2*, 216–219.

Leonard, R. J., & Kendall, K. A. (2007). *Dysphagia assessment and treatment planning: A team approach* (2nd ed.). San Diego, CA: Plural.

Murray, J. (1999). *Manual of dysphagia assessment in adults*. San Diego, CA: Singular Publishing Group.

Rosenbek, J. C., & Jones, H. N. (2009). *Dysphagia in movement disorders*. San Diego, CA: Plural.

Rosenbek, J. C., Robbins, J. A., Roecker, E. B., Coyle, J. L., & Wood, J. L. (1996). A penetration-aspiration scale. *Dysphagia, 11*, 93–98.

7 Principles of Intervention in Neuromuscular Disorders

PRINCIPLES OF TREATMENT

Once a diagnosis is made, the next question is what can be done to resolve or alleviate the problem? Intervention is at the core of rehabilitation and includes a broad range of techniques that include rehabilitative treatments designed to improve function, education about impairments, and instruction in compensatory techniques to maximize safety and/or efficiency in eating and swallowing. The reader is referred to another volume in Plural's Clinical Dysphagia Series, *Dysphagia in Movement Disorders* (Rosenbek & Jones, 2009). Here you will find six chapters devoted to intervention: Classification of Treatments, Principles of Compensatory Treatments, Principles of Rehabilitative Techniques, General Treatment Considerations, Compensatory Techniques, and Rehabilitation Techniques. This volume does not repeat what has been thoroughly described by Rosenbek and Jones as applicable to individuals with movement disorders; however, an effort is made to highlight themes that apply to neuromuscular disorders and focus attention on the differences between these two categories of impairment. Table 7–1 outlines the principles of treatment in the domains of compensation and rehabilitation as described by Rosen-

bek and Jones. Although this outline does not do justice to the depth of information that is communicated in their text, it does provide a basis for beginning a discussion of treatment as it applies to individuals with neuromuscular disorders. Furthermore, the examples and explanations provided in Table 7–1 represent an interpretation of the principles described.

Principles are universal truths and thus apply to all categories of impairment, whether movement disorders or neuromuscular. The issue is really one of selective application for a particular technique; a decision to prescribe a specific compensatory or rehabilitation technique is based on a number of factors, not the least of which is the diagnosis.

GENERAL TREATMENT CONSIDERATIONS

As discussed in depth by Rosenbek and Jones (2009), a treatment theme that cuts across the various diseases is the intent to impose some improved degree of motor control through the application of a specific technique. Improved motor control potentially can be achieved by compensatory techniques such as adjustments in posture and modifications in diet and manner of eating.

Table 7–1. Principles of Treatment for Dysphagia

Compensatory Techniques: Interventions intended for immediate impact on safety of swallowing and adequacy of nutrition and hydration

Principles	Examples and Explanations
1. A given intervention technique may have both compensatory and rehabilitative value.	Use of thickened liquids addresses the issue of safety while simultaneously allowing the individual to "exercise" swallowing.
2. Rehabilitative techniques should be used before or in concert with compensatory techniques.	Exercises designed to improve laryngeal valving are introduced for a patient needing thickened liquids to reduce risks for aspiration due to impaired vocal fold closure.
3. Compensations do not always protect patients from aspiration and its consequences	The effects of aspiration of thickened liquids are unknown and may increase the likelihood of pulmonary complications.
4. Some compensatory techniques are unacceptable to some patients.	Patients may resist postural adjustments that potentially reduce the risk of aspiration.
5. The planned duration of a prescribed compensatory technique should be considered and explained to the patient.	If the compensation is not rehabilitative and duration is likely to be for the patient's lifetime, an explanation should be provided to the patient.
6. Combinations of compensatory techniques or of compensations combined with rehabilitative techniques have the greatest likelihood for positive effect.	For a given patient, utilization of a chin tuck, head turn, and thickened liquids as compensatory techniques might be combined with laryngeal valving exercises for rehabilitation, thus providing a total therapeutic approach for the individual.
7. There is a high likelihood for noncompliance with compensatory techniques	The application of a compensatory technique should be considered in light of the likelihood for acceptance and compliance.

Rehabilitative Techniques: Intended to improve swallowing function by utilizing plasticity, or the person's ability to change experience in the domains of *muscle plasticity*, *behavioral plasticity*, and *neural plasticity*

Principles	Examples and Explanations
Muscle plasticity refers to training that is designed to increase strength or endurance by altering the chemical, cellular, and muscle fiber composition.	Requires specificity—individuals improve what they practice; therefore, treatment for swallowing should target muscular components of swallowing. Tongue exercises for protrusion and lateralization do not meet specificity requirement as these movements are not part of swallowing; whereas, tongue exercises for dorsal strength using the Iowa Oral Performance Instrument (IOPI) fulfill this principle as this motion is an important component of swallowing.

Table 7–1. *continued*

Principles	Examples and Explanations
Muscle plasticity continued	Requires overload—improvements are a consequence of exercises that require more strength and/or endurance to perform than is necessary for the normal performance of the task, in this case swallowing.
	Swallowing itself does not adequately exercise the musculature to improve strength or endurance; whereas, swallowing against resistance using something like the Masako maneuver would fulfill this principle of by providing resistance to tongue retraction.
Behavioral plasticity refers to the body's ability to alter performance through experience.	The number and spacing of repetitions of a target behavior should be considered.
	In applying traditional rehabilitative techniques for swallowing consider that: (a) massed practice may promote rapid acquisition, but submaximal retention; and (b) spaced practice tends to slow down acquisition but improves retention.
	Feedback relative to knowledge of results (KR) and knowledge of performance (KP) are important for skill learning.
	Subjective verbal feedback given to a patient by a clinician regarding the adequacy of a given behavioral response provides KR that may benefit acquisition of a target skill, whereas physiologic feedback, for example, sEMG biofeedback received during training for the Mendelsohn maneuver, may provide even more valuable KP data.
	Timing of feedback influences acquisition and retention of trained skills.
	Delayed and summary feedback that allows an individual time to self-assess performance positively influences acquisition and retention of skills when compared to immediate feedback on each trial.
Neural plasticity depends on the adaptive capacity of the central nervous system and changes in neural processes are necessary for any behavioral change.	Use it or lose it.
	There may be negative consequences for a decision to pursue non-oral nutritional support with regard to the nervous system's ability to retain a motor program for swallowing.
	Use it and improve it.
	The nervous system changes with practice and those changes will potentially improve performance.

continues

Table 7–1. *continued*	
Principles	***Examples and Explanations***

Neural plasticity continued	Specificity matters.
	  The targets for swallowing treatment should be swallowing-related movements.
	Repetition matters.
	  Multiple repetitions with optimal spacing are required to achieve desired outcomes.
	Intensity matters.
	  Optimal intensity is required to achieve the necessary neural changes for the acquisition of a skill.
	Time matters.
	  Although it is likely true that early intervention is preferable to delayed treatment, data is lacking to establish the optimal time to begin treatment.
	Salience matters.
	  Meaningful tasks are likely to be more self-reinforcing than nonmeaningful tasks; in this context, swallowing as part of eating is likely to be more powerful than nonnutrient swallows.
	Age matters.
	  Although it is easier to alter the nervous system of younger individuals, age should not influence treatment for swallowing disorders.
	Transference.
	  Although generalization has limits, treatment of one response is likely to generalize to other responses of a similar nature; for example, swallowing one bolus texture may transfer to other bolus textures.
	Interference.
	  Although neural interference has not been demonstrated in dysphagia treatment, clinicians should be aware that adjustments in swallowing behavior (e.g., maneuvers) might interfere with established patterns of swallowing.

Source: Rosenbek and Jones, 2009.

Rehabilitation techniques that attempt to facilitate motor control address the underlying impairment. In some instances a specific set of muscles may be weak; thus, muscle-strengthening exercises may be utilized. Examples include inspiratory and expiratory muscle strength training for patients with Parkinson disease (PD), or lingual strengthening, where indicated, for individuals with atypical parkinsonian syndromes or ataxia. Treatment techniques for patients with movement disorders often capitalize on a given individual's ability to impose some degree of higher level cortical control over impaired muscular systems. An example of this is the utilization of Lee Silverman Voice Therapy (LSVT) for individuals with PD and for other selected cases. LSVT, although originally targeting motor speech improvements, has been introduced as a swallowing treatment technique (El Sharkawi et al., 2002). At its foundation, LSVT requires a patient to willfully exert control over voice through vigorous, regimented training and practice. By emphasizing the concept of "think loud," the patient in effect is utilizing their retained ability to cortically drive musculature that has lost its automatic control system, for example, basal ganglia motor control. The observations of positive carryover from motor speech to swallowing appear to fulfill the principle of behavioral plasticity (see Table 7–1), but beg further investigation. A similar process of improving motor control through enhancement of cortical influence may inspire the use of a Mendelsohn maneuver, wherein swallowing is brought under conscious control by willful prolongation of laryngeal elevation. For patients with a diagnosis of the movement disorder, Wilson disease, this may be logical and effective.

For neuromuscular disorders, because of their heterogeneous nature, it is difficult to find a common theme in treatment. Here, the predominant issues of impairment relate to muscle tone, strength, and endurance. Timing of swallowing events is often disrupted due to deficits in the speed of muscle contrac-

tions and subsequent relaxation, and the incompleteness of an essential motion. Treatment must take into account the stage of the particular disease. Like the pathologic processes that cause movement disorders, neuromuscular diseases are often, but not always, degenerative in nature. For some levels of impairment, degeneration might be exceedingly slow or the disorder might even be considered to be a chronic condition, as discussed in relationship to certain forms of muscular dystrophy (MD). The typical course for other neuromuscular diseases, although still degenerative, can be quite variable, for example, myasthenia gravis (MG) and multiple sclerosis (MS). At least one neuromuscular disorder, Guillain-Barré, has a relatively favorable prognosis for partial, if not complete, recovery. Still others, particularly motor neuron diseases like amyotrophic lateral sclerosis (ALS), tend to be relentlessly progressive. Treatment approaches for neuromuscular diseases, whether compensatory or rehabilitative, must remain adaptable so as to benefit a "neurologic moving target."

Rosenbek and Jones (2009) discuss a number of "general treatment considerations" in relationship to movement disorders. These same considerations are discussed here as we view their association with neuromuscular disorders.

Team Planning

The complexity inherent in most of the diseases that fall within the neuromuscular category demands the expertise of specialists from a variety of disciplines. In most major medical centers, it is common for interdisciplinary teams to form around a diagnostic label, for example an MD clinic, MS clinic, and motor neuron disease team, to list just a few. Neuromuscular diseases affect multiple systems and can impact function in many realms: ambulation, self-care, breathing, speaking, and swallowing. Medical, surgical, prosthetic, nutritional, and pharmaceutical issues interact in ways that necessitate team communications for optimal care. Decisions regarding the nature of a treatment, the timing of its application, and the duration of its use require data from a variety of specialists. Although in all too many instances end-of-life decisions come to the fore, the burdens for patients, families, caregivers, and health professionals may be eased by team involvement.

A Combination of Techniques

As it is with movement disorders, treatment of swallowing in neuromuscular disorders often involves a combination of compensatory and rehabilitation techniques. For those with more chronic forms of dysphagia, for example individuals diagnosed with one of the milder forms of myotonic MD, a compensatory technique involving the modification of diet texture might be introduced and reinforced for lifelong application, and a rehabilitative technique of the Mendelsohn maneuver taught at a critical point in the patient's disease to bring swallowing under more conscious control. For patients with a variable disease course, as is typical for many with MG, compensatory techniques might be applicable during periods of disease exacerbation, but not needed at other times. For these individuals, any rehabilitative technique that stresses or fatigues the musculature would be contraindicated. Similarly, the variable course that is typical for patients with

relapsing-remitting MS dictates that compensations are applied during periods of exacerbation and that certain rehabilitative techniques, for example those that address inspiratory and expiratory muscle training to strengthen breathing, are used during more stable periods to help avoid complications brought on when swallowing difficulties arise.

Neuromuscular Disorders Are Often Progressive

With the exception of certain infectious and toxic muscle diseases (e.g., Lyme disease, and steroid myopathy) and infectious neuropathies (e.g., Guillain-Barré syndrome), most of the neuromuscular diseases are progressive. The rates of degeneration are variable both within and between diseases. For example, the course for a patient with the motor neuron disease progressive bulbar palsy might be very rapid and culminate in death; conversely, a patient with the motor neuron disease primary lateral sclerosis can progress slowly over 20 or more years. Because of the heterogeneous nature of these diseases, treatment decisions regarding swallowing related issues cannot be generalized. The themes that are of paramount importance and common to the treatment of swallowing in patients with degenerative neuromuscular disorders are: (1) the need to base treatment on the stage of the disease; (2) the necessity that patients have access to care provided by professionals who are knowledgeable regarding the particular disease; (3) the availability of follow-up care throughout the course of the disease; and (4) patients, families, and caregivers receive appropriate education regarding the particular condition and its management.

Reevaluation

The progressive nature of these diseases and the need for follow-up services presuppose periodic re-assessment. The frequency of reassessment will depend on the diagnosis and the unique manifestation of symptoms for an individual. For instance, systematic and thorough clinical reassessment should be relatively frequent for patients with rapidly developing or worsening symptoms, as often is the case in the motor neuron disease (ALS). Instrumental examinations, particularly radiographic swallowing studies, should be judiciously administered for patients with rapidly progressive diseases owing to issues of cost, cost-effectiveness, and risk.

Stopping Treatment

For most, though certainly not all neuromuscular disorders, maintenance of function and prevention of complications are the impetus for beginning treatment of swallowing. A decision to stop treatment can be difficult; it is difficult both for the clinician who must weigh a myriad of factors that influence the decision, and the patient who must deal with the physical and psychological consequences of a decision to stop treatment. When it is clear from available data that a treatment is not having a positive effect, whether it is compensatory or rehabilitative, it is necessary to alter course. When a treatment effect is unclear, withholding that treatment and assessing the effect might bring clarity to the situation. However, we recognize that the variable course that is typical for certain diagnoses, for example, relapsing-remitting MS, can make it challenging to determine a treatment's effectiveness vis-à-vis disease remission. Clarity of treatment goals can facilitate this decision-making process. For instance, if a patient has a rapidly progressive disease, such as ALS, the treatment goal might be to manage swallowing symptoms and minimize the risk for aspiration. Treatment duration in this example might be relatively short. However, as indicated above, a plan for periodically reconsulting to reassess and fine-tune or update management suggestions typically is indicated.

Dementia

Several of the neuromuscular diseases discussed in this volume have the potential to be complicated by cognitive decline. Frontotemporal dementia is found in certain presentations of ALS. Patients with MS can experience cognitive problems and these can be complicating factors in certain forms of MD. Measuring cognitive capabilities and tracking patients for changes is critical when considering the application of both compensatory and rehabilitative techniques for treatment of swallowing. When dementia is a factor, or even when milder cognitive decline is present, caregiver training is necessary. Caregiver-controlled application of a treatment intervention, although generally less effective than patient-directed behaviors, can be beneficial and treatment should not automatically be dismissed when cognitive issues are evident.

Tube Feeding

Although there are guidelines for instituting tube feedings for some neuromuscular diseases, particularly a percutaneous endoscopic gastrostomy (PEG) for patients with ALS (Miller et al., 2009), it is clinical judgment that is required to decide when this topic should be broached. Misconceptions and misinformation abound around the topic of feeding tubes. When introducing a discussion about tube feeding, it is important to recognize the following:

1. Tube feeding does not preclude some oral feeding. In some cases, a patient might take primary nutrition via a PEG and oral intake for pleasure, or primary nutrition orally and PEG feeding for nutritional or hydration supplementation. Others rely on tube feeding only during periods of disease exacerbation and take full oral nutrition at other times.

2. Treatment can be ongoing even after the placement of a PEG. It is not uncommon for a feeding tube placement to be initiated in advance of need. For example, patients who have declining respiratory functions in combination with a swallowing impairment might be wise to undergo the PEG procedure while they are still able to breathe and tolerate the procedure comfortably. In general, PEG placement is optimally performed before a patient reaches nutritional crisis.

3. Feeding tubes can positively impact quality of life by stabilizing nutritional intake, improving energy, eliminating time-pressure associated with eating, and reducing fear associated with choking. In some instances, maintaining adequate nutritional support can also aid slowing of disease progression.

4. Tube feeding does not prevent aspiration and, for some, can increase the risk. Precautions instituted for those patients not taking nutrition orally include the institution of meticulous oral care to reduce the likelihood of lung contamination from oral microbes and instruction to maintain an upright posture during and following feedings to reduce the risk of gastroesophageal reflux and aspiration.

5. Patients are likely to view the placement of a feeding tube as an end-of-life decision. It is essential that education and counseling directed to patients and their families clarify a feeding tube's purpose; that the potential benefits relative to the patient's enhanced physical status and quality of life are clearly articulated.

Impaired Judgment

A patient's denial and/or minimization of swallowing impairment is not uncommon for those with a neuromuscular disease. When there is uncertainty regarding a patient's status, careful clinical assessment of the neuromuscular mechanism and instrumental measures of the biomechanics of swallowing are needed for documentation. Data derived from family and caregiver reports are critically important in the assessment process. Dependence on others for support during feeding is also reality for many individuals. Recognizing the need for support and demonstrating techniques that optimize the feeding process is critical to successful treatment.

Comorbidity

Coexisting conditions are more the rule than the exception for patients with neuromuscular diseases. There is no recognizable pattern for the particular conditions that could be impacting swallowing at any given point in time. Clearly, neuromuscular diseases are predisposed to impair multiple muscular systems, most commonly respiration and limb functions. Whenever a disease is severely disabling and mobility is limited, patients are more susceptible to conditions related to a sedentary life and these can potentially lead to issues of organ failure and skin breakdown. In addition, certain additional diagnoses, for example, gastroesophageal reflux, may exacerbate the existing dysphagia. Swallowing treatment must be viewed in light of these possibilities and clinicians must be cognizant of the patient's priorities for treatment and controlling for additional contributing factors.

Other Considerations

Rosenbek and Jones (2009) have indicated that for patients with movement disorders there is a tendency to refer for treatment of behavioral symptoms only after medical and surgical interventions have been exhausted. This is not as consistently the case with neuromuscular disease. The most common forms of pathology at the level of muscle, myopathy, are genetically based and there is little in the way of medical and surgical intervention that can address the impairment. For these patients, treatment of dysphagia tends to be addressed as symptoms appear. Impairment at the neuromuscular junction, most typically MG, is often managed longterm by pharmacologic interventions and these can be effective in preventing or delaying the onset of behavioral symptoms, including dysphagia. There are situations where referral for treatment of dysphagia is delayed, but well-informed health care practitioners recognize the benefit of early intervention by a specialist in swallowing disorders. When neuromuscular pathology occurs at the levels of the motor neurons, as in ALS, or the myelinated axons of the CNS, as with MS, medical and surgical treatment is quite limited. In these situations, it is ideal if the dysphagia specialist is an integral partner in team treatment, such that there is an opportunity to address the symptoms from the moment they are recognized. It is critical that health care professionals are educated and informed regarding the importance of timely referrals for patients with neuromuscular disorders because effective treatment is often available to prevent the devastating consequences of unattended dysphagia.

CRITICAL FACTORS IN DEVELOPING A TREATMENT PLAN

There are several important factors to consider in developing an effective treatment plan for patients with neuromuscular disorders. These include: (1) diagnosis and prognosis, (2) the International Classification of Functioning, Disability and Health, (3) evidence-based practice—benefits and limits, (4) estimated cost-benefit, and (5) patient preferences and values.

Diagnosis and Prognosis

Knowledge of the medical/neurologic diagnosis is fundamental to effective intervention. In a clinical setting, patients may present with a variety of differing neurological diagnoses. Add to this, a variety of underlying medical conditions or risk factors, and it becomes apparent that there is no single approach that will be appropriate or effective for every patient. Clinical hypotheses regarding the nature of the dysphagia are developed based on this information, and tested through the process of the clinical swallowing exam (see Chapter 4). This information, considered within the context of what is known or theorized about normal and disordered neurologic functioning and swallowing, is critical to development of appropriate and effective intervention.

Knowledge of the underlying medical and neurologic diagnoses, and the specific neuromuscular and biomechanical dysphagia diagnosis, will shed light on the issue of prognosis. Prognosis is a judgment of what will be the most likely outcome for a particular patient. This judgment is determined based on research examining outcomes for particular conditions and clinical experience. It is important to acknowledge, however, that evidence-based prognosis determinations for groups of people tend to be more accurate than for individuals. Due to the large number of potential variables, it is never possible to predict with 100% accuracy the outcome for an individual. Put another way, prognostic statements given to patients are often based on statistical averages taken for a group, and we should not treat a patient like a statistical average. Nevertheless, prognosis must be taken into consideration in planning intervention. For instance, it is well known that ALS is a degenerative disease with progressive disintegration of muscular function. Therefore, in the treatment of a person with ALS and significant dysphagia, in most instances it does not make sense to write a goal targeting return to "normal" swallowing function.

Both diagnosis and prognosis are important considerations. Taken together, this information provides a basis for determining what will be the most effective intervention plan for a given patient.

International Classification of Functioning, Disability, and Health

When developing an intervention plan, it is important to consider how to measure its effectiveness. Historically, the most used intervention outcomes for swallowing and communication disorders have been based on measurement of impairments. A problem with use of impairment-based measures in tracking outcomes associated with rehabilitation is that these measures do not take into account success with management or compensation for impairments, nor do they measure one's functioning in the real world. Speech-language pathologists were among the first to observe this discrepancy with outcomes for persons with aphasia, and the first to develop the concept of functional skills (Taylor, 1965).

The International Classification of Functioning, Disability and Health (ICF) is a biopsychosocial model focused on human function as opposed to disability, and participation as opposed to handicap. This model, outlined in Figure 7–1, acknowledges differing components of functioning. In addition to changes to body structure and function, commonly thought of as the impairment, the ICF distinguishes activity, as one's ability to execute an action or task, and participation, defined as involvement in life situations. The ICF model acknowledges the dynamic and complex interactions that can occur between functioning and con-

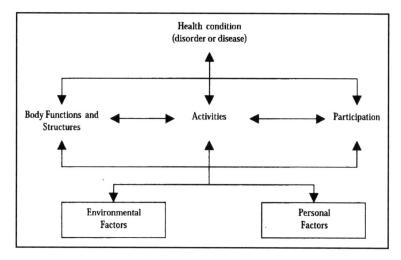

Figure 7–1. International Classification of Functioning, Disability and Health (ICF) http://www.worldenable.net/escapstats/p resentationwhoicfintro.htm ("Towards a Common Language for Functioning, Disability and Health: ICF [The International Classification of Functioning, Disability and Health]," 2002). Used with permission.

textual factors, such as the environment and the person's internal perception. Therefore, this model provides a construct to aid in the assessment of the success of various rehabilitation interventions, including swallowing treatment.

Consider a patient with ALS and mild-moderate oropharyngeal dysphagia; as ALS is progressive, it is unlikely that intervention will result in significant improvements at the impairment level, that is, no improvement in body structure and function. However, patient education about dysphagia, along with use of compensatory strategies, can greatly improve a patient's comfort with eating modified textures and allow the patient to participate with certain aspects of eating despite the impairment. If the clinician tracks impairments only to indicate intervention outcomes, it will appear that intervention has had no effect. Therefore, tracking the effect of interventions at the level of activities and participation becomes critical.

It is also important to acknowledge the impact of contextual factors, that is, environmental and personal factors, on the outcome. For instance, many treatment strategies manipulate the environment, for example, eliminating distractions during meals, or modify the bolus by changing the temperature of foods. Dysphagia scales, such as the SWAL-QOL (McHorney et al., 2002) and EAT-10 (Belafsky et al., 2008), aid the swallowing clinician's ability to assess and monitor outcomes and the effectiveness of interventions related to the activity and participation aspects of swallowing.

Evidence-Based Practice and Levels of Evidence

Over the past two decades, an increased focus has been placed on the importance of evidence-based practice. Recently, this effort has increased. For instance, the journal *Neurology* has determined that all therapeutic clinical trials submitted will be required to include a level of evidence (LOE) classification. The LOE classification scheme developed and used by American Academy of Neurology (AAN) for purposes of judging therapeutic interventions is detailed in Tables 7–2 and 7–3

Table 7–2. American Academy of Neurology (AAN) Classification of Evidence for Therapeutic Intervention

Class I: Prospective, randomized, controlled clinical trial with masked outcome assessment, in a representative population. The following are required:
  a) primary outcome(s) clearly defined
  b) exclusion/inclusion criteria clearly defined
  c) adequate accounting for dropouts and crossovers with numbers sufficiently low to have minimal potential for bias
  d) relevant baseline characteristics are presented and substantially equivalent among treatment groups or there is appropriate statistical adjustment for differences

Class II: Prospective matched group cohort study in a representative population with masked outcome assessment that meets a to d above OR a RCT in a representative population that lacks one criteria in (*a*) to (*d*).

Class III: All other controlled trials (including well-defined natural history controls or patients serving as own controls) in a representative population, where outcome is independently assessed, or independently derived by objective outcome measurement.

Class IV: Evidence from uncontrolled studies, case series, case reports, or expert opinion.

Table 7–3. AAN Classification of Recommendations

A = Established as effective, ineffective or harmful (or established as useful/predictive or not useful/predictive) for the given condition in the specified population. (Level A rating requires at least two consistent Class I studies.)

B = Probably effective, ineffective, or harmful (or probably useful/predictive or not useful/predictive) for the given condition in the specified population. (Level B rating requires at least one Class I study or two consistent Class II studies.)

C = Possibly effective, ineffective, or harmful (or possibly useful/predictive or not useful/predictive) for the given condition in the specified population. (Level C rating requires at least one Class II study or two consistent Class III studies.)

U = Data inadequate or conflicting; given current knowledge, treatment (test, predictor) is unproven.

(Edlund, Gronseth, So, & Franklin, 2004). The American Congress of Rehabilitation Medicine Clinical Practice Committee has also adopted the AAN classification as their preferred method for developing clinical guidelines (Johnston, Sherer, & Whyte, 2006).

Benefits

There clearly are some benefits in use of levels of evidence classification schemes. The criteria are clearly stated and aid the ability of organizations, researchers, and clinicians to systematically review current literature on particular intervention topics. These and other criteria raise the bar with respect to encouraging well-designed studies to address topics relevant to therapy and other forms of intervention, such as pharmacologic treatments. Individual practitioners are better able to assess potential intervention techniques with regard to potential risk and benefit. In its best implementation, evidence-based practice is the integration of an individual practitioner's clinical expertise with the best clinical evidence arising from systematic research (Sackett, Rosenberg, Gray, Haynes, & Richardson, 1996). As it currently stands, LOE criteria tend to be applied more successfully to "medical" issues, that is, research with the goal of reducing pathology or impairment level conditions, than to behavioral or psychosocial interventions (Johnston et al., 2006).

Limits

Although there clearly are many benefits to the currently established classification schemes toward the goals of evidence-based practice, several caveats should be acknowledged (Johnston et al., 2006):

Limited Availability of Evidence. Evidence is useful and should be considered, if it exists. Experienced clinicians know, however, that clinically applicable evidence in the literature is frequently sparse and incomplete. Currently, there is a paucity of research examining intervention topics for dysphagia as it applies to many neurologic diseases. Furthermore, often studies with negative results are not submitted or not accepted for publication.

Bias in Published Research. The availability of research on any topic is dependent on the level of funding to support the research. It also is dependent on the pattern for acceptance of submissions for publication. Research literature is frequently biased due to tendencies to publish on topics that are both well funded and report positive results.

Statistical Versus Clinical Significance. Findings of statistical significance on intervention studies do not always clearly indicate the clinical significance. Clinical significance can be determined by a variety of factors, for example, magnitude or strength of the treatment effect, importance of the clinical question, and personal characteristics of individual patients. Ottenbacher (1995) stated this problem well: "It is a mistake to equate statistical significance with practical or clinical significance. Statistical results, from even the best designed experimental trials, can overestimate or underestimate clinical importance." It is important to note that statistical significance does not indicate magnitude of effect; it only indicates whether or not the null hypothesis was determined to be true. In addition, statistical significance can be manipulated by factors such as the study design and sample size.

Study design. The gold-standard randomized controlled trial (RCT) study design may not work as well for some rehabilitation, behavioral-based treatments, as it does for drug studies. It is a challenge to isolate and define all of the therapeutic factors that are involved when complex, multifaceted approaches to treatment are being employed. Additionally, outcomes for rehabilitation are multidimensional and calculated in terms of physiological change, social participation and well-being, which make measurement and analysis complex.

Practical and Ethical Considerations for RCTs. In most instances, randomized placebo-controlled trials would be considered unethical in the rehabilitation setting. For example, employing a "substitute intervention" for acute onset dysphagia that might delay functional recovery puts the patient at risk for serious medical complications. It obviously would be unethical to withhold many of the currently available interventions targeting swallowing safety to prove their effectiveness.

Concluding Thoughts

For the reasons cited above, it is important to have a balanced perspective vis-à-vis the employment of principles of evidence-based practice. However, it is equally important to have a solid rationale for proposed interventions from the perspective of current knowledge of normal and disordered neurologic and swallowing function, as indicated in the section above. It is essential to use clinical common sense, based on experience and professional knowledge of the normal neuromuscular system and what is known about the patient's diagnoses, in addition to consideration of current published evidence.

Estimated Cost-Benefit

For most patients there are limits that are placed on their healthcare benefits. Reimbursement schemes applied for rehabilitation services have varied greatly from time to time. Often, rehabilitation services have a lifetime limit and, therefore, cost-benefit estimates enter into the equation of determining whether or not to provide treatment at any particular point in time. If expensive equipment is to be utilized in a rehabilitative strategy, the cost-benefit ratio is a critical factor, as are diagnosis and LOE.

Patient Preference and Values

Patient adherence to recommendations is a major issue in swallowing treatment. Despite providing the most well-informed advice and most efficacious interventions, there will be times when carryover and follow-through with recommendations is poor. Within the context of rehabilitation, treatment goals should accommodate patient goals. To this end, goals should be negotiated with the patient. However, even when the patient is in agreement with the goal and has the good intention to implement recommendations, there are times when the patient does not follow through. This can happen for a number of reasons that include: inability to initiate, poor recall of recommendations, ambivalence regarding advice, or a conscious choice to ignore or delay implementation. For instance, many patients make a quality of life choice to continue eating despite aspiration risk. If a patient decides not to follow through with recommendations, should he or she then be labeled noncompliant and treatment efforts abandoned? These issues are controversial, but especially relevant in the realm of degenerative diseases and end-of-life choices.

Per the ethical principle of fidelity, the clinician should not abandon the patient even in the face of willful noncompliance. Attitudes and circumstances change, especially for patients with degenerative diseases, and a period of noncompliance can be a manifestation of the adjustment and coping processes. Noncompliance also may simply reflect the patient's personal preference or choice. In accordance with the ethical principle of autonomy, individual patients should be afforded their rights with respect to decision making regarding their own care. The clinician can support the process of informed decision making through efforts to educate patients regarding the rationale for stated recommendations.

Motivation is key. Even for willful or noncompliant patients, it has been shown that for many health conditions offering a diagnosis and advising on recommendations is frequently insufficient for effecting change in behavior. Individually planned counseling becomes an important component of intervention toward the goal of enhancing patient motivation for change, which in turn can result in improved compliance with recommendations. Counseling may serve the additional purpose of educating the patient to aid informed decision-making. Motivational interviewing is an example of an effective counseling approach that has been shown to be effective in improving motivation and

enthusiasm to follow through with a variety of health recommendations (Bundy, 2004). The motivational interviewing approach can be applied to counseling in relation to swallowing intervention. However, counseling techniques such as this require awareness and training of the clinician. Table 7–4 presents an overview of the concepts underlying motivational interviewing.

Even the most persuasive clinician using powerful motivational counseling techniques will encounter patients who are aware and clear in their expression of a preference that is contrary to sound clinical recommendations. In these instances, it is possible to balance recommendations and accommodation of patient preferences. First, it is important to educate the patient regarding the therapeutic diagnosis and rationale for recommendations. This education empowers the patient so that he or she can make an informed decision about how they wish to proceed. If the patient expresses a preference that is contrary to the recommendations, the clinician should respond by acknowledging and documenting the patient's preference, along with further education to ensure that the recommendations were clearly understood. When it is clear that the patient is informed of risks associated with their decision, a clinician may then offer suggestions for alternative ways of minimizing risks that are in line with the patient's preference. For example, if thickened liquids are recommended for a patient and the patient indicates they will not adhere to this recommendation, you can then complete further education on the risk for aspiration associated with this choice and discuss other ways to minimize the aspiration risk should the patient continue with thin liquids.

Table 7–4. Principles of Motivational Interviewing

Express empathy: This involves active listening, acceptance, and reflection of what the patient has conveyed. This helps to resolve ambivalence about change.

Example: "I hear and truly understand that you do not like the idea of a supplemental feeding tube."

Roll with resistance/avoid argument: Argument is rehearsal of reasons to avoid change, and is therefore counterproductive. Resistance should not be directly opposed by the clinician. Rather, the clinician interprets resistance as a signal to respond differently.

Example:

Clinician: "Tell me why you are not using nectar thick liquids?"

Patient: "Well, I have been drinking nectar thick liquids sometimes! They taste terrible though!"

Clinician: "OK, it sounds like you have genuinely tried to modify your diet. Perhaps we can discuss ideas for making this adjustment more palatable."

Support self-efficacy: Encourage and draw out overt positive statements regarding the possibility of change from the patient's perspective. Assist with reframing negative statements to be more positive. The clinician works to enhance the patient's self-confidence.

Example:

Patient: "I tried the recommended exercises, but it was too difficult."

Clinician: "It is great that you remembered the recommendation and put forth energy to try them out. Let's discuss exactly what happened and let me hear any ideas you might have."

Develop discrepancy: Elicit goals from the patient. Develop awareness of the current situation and consequences. Identify differences between the current and ideal situation. Change is then motivated by the discrepancy between the patient's valued goals and the present behavior. The patient (not the clinician) should indicate the reasons for change.

Example:

Clinician: "Tell me about your concerns."

Patient: "I would like to be able to eat regular foods again."

Clinician: "Let me show you the results of your swallowing study . . . We can see that your airway protection is better when you are in a neck flexion position. When your chin is tilted upward, you aspirated."

Patient: "OK, so I will be able to swallow better in the chin-down position."

Source: Bundy, 2004; Medley and Powell, 2010.

SUMMARY

Intervention is at the core of rehabilitation. Intervention is multifaceted and may include education about impairments, treatments designed to improve function, instruction in management techniques for safety, and/or instruction in compensatory strategies. Consideration of diagnosis, prognosis, functional goals (including activities and participation), evidence-based practice, and patient values are important in developing an effective treatment plan.

REFERENCES

Belafsky, P. C., Mouadeb, D. A., Rees, C. J., Pryor, J. C., Postma, G. N., Allen, J., & Leonard, R. J. (2008). Validity and reliability of the Eating Assessment Tool (EAT-10). *Annals of Otology, Rhinology and Laryngology, 117*(12), 919–924.

Bundy, C. (2004). Changing behaviour: Using motivational interviewing techniques. *Journal of the Royal Society of Medicine, 97*(Suppl. 44), 43–47.

Edlund, W., Gronseth, G., So, Y., & Franklin, G. (2004). *Clinical practice guideline process manual.* St. Paul, MN: American Academy of Neurology.

El Sharkawi, A., Ramig, L., Logemann, J. A., Pauloski, B. R., Rademaker, A. W., Smith, C. H., . . . Werner, C. (2002). Swallowing and voice effects of Lee Silverman Voice Treatment (LSVT®): A pilot study. *Journal of Neurology, Neurosurgery, and Psychiatry, 72*, 31–36.

Johnston, M. V., Sherer, M., & Whyte, J. (2006). Applying evidence standards to rehabilitation research. *American Journal of Physical Medicine and Rehabilitation, 85*(4), 292–309.

McHorney, C. A., Robbins, J., Lomax, K., Rosenbek, J. C., Chignell, K., & Kramer, A. E., (2002). The SWAL-QOL and SWAL-CARE outcomes tool for oropharyngeal dysphagia in adults: III. Documentation of reliability and validity. *Dysphagia, 17*(2), 97–114.

Medley, A. R., & Powell, T. (2010). Motivational Interviewing to promote self-awareness and engagement in rehabilitation following acquired brain injury: A conceptual review. *Neuropsychology Rehabilitation, 20*, 481–508.

Miller, R. G., Jackson, C. E., Kasarskis, E. J., England, J. D., Forshew, D., Johnston, W., . . . Woolley, S. C. (2009). Practice Parameter update: The care of the patient with amyotrophic lateral sclerosis: Drug, nutritional, and respiratory therapies (an evidence-based review). *Neurology, 73*, 1218–1226.

Ottenbacher, K. J. (1995). Why rehabilitation research does not work (as well as we think it should). *Archives of Physical Medicine and Rehabilitation, 76*(2), 123–129.

Rosenbek, J. C., & Jones, H. N. (2009). *Dysphagia in movement disorders.* San Diego, CA: Plural.

Sackett, D. L., Rosenberg, W. M., Gray, J. A., Haynes, R. B., & Richardson, W. S. (1996). Evidence-based medicine: What it is and what it isn't. *British Medical Journal, 312*(7023), 71–72.

Taylor, M. L. (1965). A measure of functional communication in aphasia. *Archives of Physical Medicine and Rehabilitation,* 101–107.

Towards a common language for functioning, disability and health: ICF (The International Classification of Functioning, Disability and Health). *British Medical Journal* (2002). Geneva, Switzerland: ICF.

8 Muscle Disease

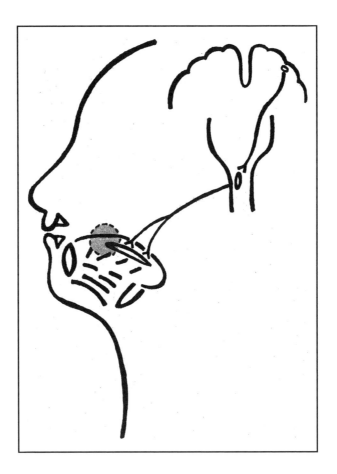

MYOPATHY

The term *myopathy* is the designation for a disease that affects muscle fibers, as opposed to nerves, and impacts muscles connected to bones, that is, skeletal muscles. A myopathy may be caused by an inherited genetic defect (e.g., muscular dystrophies), autoimmune inflammation (e.g., dermatomyositis), endocrine disorder (e.g., hyperthyroidism), metabolic disorder (e.g., glycogen storage disease), and/or toxic condition (e.g., excessive alcohol).

The symptoms of myopathy are somewhat limited because muscles have a narrow range of possible reactions that include weakness, aching, cramping, pain, tenderness, and stiffness. Typically, muscles affected by myopathy will atrophy, or waste away; however, there are notable exceptions found in certain forms of inherited myotonia in which muscles enlarge or hypotrophy.

Histology of muscles affected by myopathy generally shows nonspecific changes. The common pathologies found on muscle biopsy include muscle fiber necrosis, evidence of muscle fiber regeneration, increases in muscle connective tissue, and structural abnormalities such as nuclei changes. In certain instances, however, the histological changes in muscle tissue will have diagnostic significance. For example, abnormal fibrous rod formations found within muscle cells are indicative of *nemaline myopathy*, a nonprogressive condition causing delayed motor development, significant respiratory impairment, and involvement of the arms, legs, trunk, pharyngeal, and facial muscles.

Classification of Myopathies

There is no generally accepted classification system for all myopathies. Various specialists who have studied muscle diseases have proposed detailed classifications for inflammatory myopathies, inherited types of disease, metabolic and endocrine disorders, and toxic etiologies for myopathy. Some have used an approach to classification that focused on the pathologic features of the disease, whereas others have used clinical features or etiology to categorize the disorders. In almost all classification systems there are overlapping features; that is, a particular disease or condition might be found in more than one category (e.g., hyperthyroidism is an endocrine-based disorder that produces a toxin-induced myopathy), and the same underlying etiology may be found in both congenital and acquired forms. The following list is adapted from several sources and is offered to help clinicians involved with diagnosing and treating dysphagia to develop an overview of myopathies:

- Neurogenic myopathies—resulting from either muscle denervation or disuse atrophy
- Infectious myopathies—some have known infectious agents such as viruses, bacteria, fungus, and parasites; specific causes include trichinosis, toxoplasmosis, human immunodeficiency virus (HIV), coxsackie A and B viruses, influenza, Lyme disease, and *Staphylococcus aureus* muscle infection
- Autoimmune inflammatory myopathies—also classified as idiopathic myopathies, they generally include polymyositis, dermatomyositis, and juvenile myositis, with certain forms of inclusion body myositis having an autoimmune component; systemic lupus erythematosus, rheumatoid arthritis, and polyarteritis nodosa are idiopathic myopathies associated with connective tissue disease
- Other inflammatory myopathies—includes both sporadic inclusion body myositis (sIBM) and hereditary inclusion body myopathy (hIBM), with sIBM having some autoimmune processes involved in the pathology

- Endocrine disorders—myopathies associated with adrenal gland dysfunction such as Cushing disease and steroid myopathy, the most common endocrine myopathy; thyroid disorders of hypothyroidism (myxedema) or hyperthyroidism (e.g., Graves disease and thyrotoxic myopathy); parathyroid dysfunction, as found in multiple endocrine neoplasia; pituitary gland dysfunction, either hypopituitary or hyperpituitary disease; and pancreatic impairment associated with islets of Langerhans dysfunction causing diabetic myopathy
- Metabolic disorders—a group of well-defined genetically based impairments in metabolism caused by specific enzymatic defects; classified as a glycogen storage disease (marked by impairments in muscle cell membrane permeability that limits the transport of glucose into the muscle), lipid storage disease (errors in the production of nutrients that help the body turn fat into the energy needed for sustained exercise), and disorders of purine nucleotide metabolism (impairments in the enzymatic transformation of molecules found within muscle tissue into organic compounds that store and provide energy for high-intensity exercise of short duration)
- Toxic conditions—drug induced myopathies with a variety of toxic affects on muscle include the following: steroids (also categorized as an endocrine-based myopathy), statins (used to lower plasma cholesterol levels), alcohol (chronic alcohol abuse is known to cause striated skeletal muscle alcoholic myopathy characterized by marked weakness), cocaine (and other illicit drugs such as amphetamines, heroin, and phencyclidine or PCP), antiretroviral drugs (commonly used to treat HIV), colchicine (a natural product with toxic effects used to treat rheumatic complaints, especially gout), and antimalarials
- Hypokalemic myopathy—abnormalities in blood potassium level (including hyperkalemia) produce an electrolyte imbalance that interferes with the nervous system's ability to conduct neural impulses to muscles; hypokalemia is the most common cause of acute periodic paralysis and may be brought on by excessive fluid loss due to diarrhea, vomiting, sweating, diuretic drugs, kidney disease, eating disorders, or the ingestion of large amounts of licorice
- Inherited genetic defects—a large category that includes all forms of muscle disorders that are either present at birth or have a genetic basis and may be further delineated as a congenital myopathy or muscular dystrophy
  - Congenital myopathies—inherited disorders characterized by microscopic changes in muscles that contribute to a loss of tone and weakness in infancy, but without degenerative changes that imply a gradual decline in muscle strength and bulk; the five most common are: (1) nemaline myopathy, (2) myotubular myopathy, (3) central core myopathy, (4) congenital fiber type disproportion, and (5) multicore myopathy
  - Muscular dystrophies—inherited disorders in which there is a

dystrophic (degenerative) process causing gradual decline in strength and muscle bulk (see discussion below for details)

The inflammatory myopathies, particularly inclusion body myositis, polymyositis, and dermatomyositis, can have a major negative impact on swallowing. These diseases can impair components of the pharyngeal and esophageal phases of swallowing. For patients with inclusion body myositis, dysphagia is often a presenting symptom (Wintzen, Bots, de Bakker, Hulshof, & Padberg, 1988) and can occur at a rate of 80% (Houser, Calabrese, & Stone, 1998). For these patients, dysphagia is considered to be a progressive condition and can lead to major respiratory complications and even death due to aspiration (Oh, Brumfield, Hoskin, Kasperbauer, & Basford, 2008). In polymyositis and dermatomyositis dysphagia is also highly prevalent. Striated muscles of the pharynx and upper esophagus are commonly impaired, with specific evidence of cricopharyngeal sphincter impairment (Dalakas & Hohlfeld, 2003). These patients, if not readily identified and properly managed, can be at high risk for complications associated with aspiration.

MUSCULAR DYSTROPHIES

Definition

Muscular dystrophy (MD) is not a single condition, but a collection of more than 30 genetically based disorders characterized by weakness and progressive degeneration of muscle tissue. These inherited disorders may be recognized during infancy or later, even into adulthood. The pathology of MD can be identified in the involved muscles themselves; therefore, the impairment is considered to be a muscular disorder and not strictly neuromuscular. However, because the nature of the clinical presentation in many patients with MD is similar to that of patients with neuromuscular disease, they are described here as a pathology at the level of the muscle fibers.

It also is important to recognize that there may be some secondary involvement of at least the peripheral nervous system in certain patients with MD. Although definitive evidence is lacking, EMG and nerve conduction studies are often abnormal and point to a possible concomitant peripheral nerve impairment (Quijano-Roy et al., 2004). One possible basis for this combination of pathologies may be found in the mutation of certain proteins, laminins, which are important for both peripheral nerve and muscle development. Dystrophic mice, for example, demonstrate pathology in both peripheral nerves and muscles (Yu, Yu, & Chen, 2007). Additionally, neurologic symptoms such as cognitive impairments and apathy are found in some patients with MD, more commonly in certain forms of the disorder, for example, myotonic dystrophy. More details regarding the various symptoms of MD are described in following outline of the nine commonly recognized categories:

1. Duchenne muscular dystrophy (DMD)
   - Overview—It is considered the most severe form of MD and usually begins with progressive weakness and atrophy of leg and pelvic muscles, but also may involve arms, neck, and other skeletal muscles.
   - Occurrence—DMD primarily affects males, with a less

severe form found in females. Considered to be the most common form of MD, it occurs in approximately 1 out of every 3,600 male births.

- Course—Symptoms usually are apparent before age 6 and the ability to walk is often lost by age 12.
- Pathology—DMD is most commonly inherited in an autosomal recessive pattern where the mutated gene is received from each parent. The defective gene is responsible for the production of dystrophin, a protein that is essential for the development of normal muscle cell structures.
- Complications—Cardiomyopathy, heart arrhythmias, muscular and skeletal deformities (including macroglossia), and pulmonary symptoms including pneumonia and respiratory failure are possible complications.
- Cognition—Boys with DMD generally have lower scores on cognitive performance scales and mental retardation is possible (Hinton, De Vivo, Nereo, Goldstein, & Stern, 2000).
- Swallowing—Dysphagia is not uncommon in DMD and may become a greater problem with advancing age. Pharyngeal stage abnormalities such as vallecular and pyriform sinus residue and poor pharyngeal stripping are found more commonly in patients reaching their 20s (Nozaki et al., 2007), but even patients in their teens have been found to have laryngeal penetration without aspiration (Aloysius et al., 2008).

Hanayama and associates (2008) reported that 71% of DMD patients in their teens cough when eating, with 97% showing radiographic abnormalities on swallow studies. Pane and colleagues (2006) studied over 100 patients with DMD and also noted that patients generally took longer to eat with increasing age. However, in contrast to other the other studies, they report that choking and other clinical signs of dysphagia are less frequent after age 18 and that aspiration pneumonia was very infrequent, occurring in only 7 of 118 patients. Many patients with DMD require tracheostomy and mechanical ventilation. Although tracheostomy generally is considered to be an impediment to swallowing, a recent study has shown that invasive ventilation via tracheostomy may actually improve certain parameters of swallowing (Terzi et al., 2010).

2. Becker muscular dystrophy (BMD)
   - Overview—This inherited disease has a male distribution pattern and clinical presentation that is quite similar to DMD, but generally is milder and has a later onset of symptoms. There are generally delayed gross motor milestones with evidence of progressive and symmetric proximal muscle weakness and atrophy. Enlarged calves also may be evident.
   - Occurrence—BMD affects older boys and young men and occurs in approximately 1 in 30,000 male births.

- Course—The mean age of onset is 11 years, with a range of 2 to 21 years. Patients generally become nonambulatory between the ages of 12 to 30 years.
- Pathology—BMD, like DMD, is caused by a failure to produce the protein dystrophin, but in this case the disease is inherited in an autosomal dominant pattern (only one parent is required to transmit the abnormal gene). For DMD, dystrophin levels have been measured at less than 5% of normal, whereas in BMD the levels are generally within 30 to 80% of normal (Angelini et al., 1994).
- Complications—Respiratory impairments and cardiomyopathy are present in a majority of cases, and for some these might be the first sign of BMD. Those with early onset of symptoms are more likely to develop cardiac symptoms. Although some experience a normal life span, death from complications can occur from about age 40. Deformities such as kyphosis and contractures at the elbow may also be present and occur in later life.
- Cognition—Impairments in cognitive functions for patients with BMD have been described as less severe than those with DMD. However, some BMD patients do have nonprogressive cognitive problems. Furthermore, there is evidence that the presence of mental impairments may be related to the location of the gene deletion for both patients with DMD and BMD (Giliberto, Ferreiro, Dalamon, & Szijan, 2004).
- Swallowing—Impairments in swallowing have not been specifically studied in patients with BMD. However, given that the underlying pathology is similar to that of patients with DMD, it is likely that the same characteristics and difficulties with swallowing might be found in these patients, although perhaps in a milder form and developing later in life. With the common occurrence of respiratory impairment in patients with BMD, this feature may also contribute to impaired swallow functions.

3. Emery-Dreifuss muscular dystrophy (EDMD)
   - Overview—EDMD affects boys by causing symmetric weakness in the shoulders and upper arms and early-onset of disabling contractures at the elbow, spine, and ankle. Abnormalities of cardiac function stemming from abnormalities in the way electrical signals control the heartbeat are common and can cause syncope. Placement of a pacemaker is often necessary.
   - Occurrence—This is a rare disease estimated to occur in about 1 case per 100,000.
   - Course—There generally is slow development of contractures and weakness, which can become evident at any time from infancy to the third decade of life, with the teen years the most common time of onset. Cardiac symptoms are manifested between the teen years and the age of 40.
   - Pathology—The cause is attributed to mutations of genes responsible for the production

of the protein emerin and other proteins that surround the nucleus of each muscle cell. It may be inherited in an autosomal dominant or recessive pattern.

- Complications—Many of the complications associated with EDMD are related to the cardiac impairments and muscle contractures. For example, sudden cardiac death is not uncommon. A stiff neck, toe walking, and a "waddling gait" are frequently described.
- Cognition—Delays in the development of mental functions and cognitive impairments associated with EDMD have not been reported.
- Swallowing—Specific impairments in swallowing and other functions associated with facial and oral-pharyngeal musculature have not been identified.

4. Limb-girdle muscular dystrophy (LGMD)
   - Overview—Considered to be a group of disorders, as opposed to a single disease, LGMD affects both men and women in equal numbers. It causes weakness and atrophy of proximal muscles, especially around the hips and shoulders. Given that there are many genetic subtypes of the disease, misdiagnosis is common.
   - Occurrence—Because this is such a heterogeneous condition with a lack of diagnostic specificity, there are few reports of prevalence and estimates are not helpful.
   - Course—Slowly developing symptoms begin to become apparent in late childhood to

early adulthood. Those with earlier onset of symptoms are more likely to progress faster and the weakness becomes more disabling. Although not a fatal disease, those with heart involvement are at risk for secondary complications.

- Pathology—At least 15 separate genes and hundreds of different mutations have been implicated in the various forms of LGMD, which can be inherited in either a dominant or recessive pattern. Many of these genes are responsible for the production of proteins that are located in muscle cell membranes. Missing or diminished proteins lead to muscles that are more susceptible to injury from the normal contraction and relaxation cycles.
- Complications—Cardiac impairments of cardiomyopathy, conduction abnormalities and arrhythmias are possible, but not as common as in some other forms of MD. Respiratory function decline is also possible in certain forms of this disease.
- Cognition—Impairments in intellectual functions and sensory modalities are not implicated in LGMD.
- Swallowing—Impairments in swallowing and other facial-oral-pharyngeal functions are not associated with LGMD.

5. Facioscapulohumeral muscular dystrophy (FSH) or Landouzy-Dejerine disease
   - Overview—One of the most common presentations of MD, FSH begins in late childhood to early adulthood with weakness in facial muscles, particularly

around the lips and eyes, and weakness and wasting around the shoulders and upper arms. Hips and lower extremities are affected in some individuals. There frequently is loss of muscle tissue in affected areas. The involvement of facial muscles often leads to misinterpretation of facial expression, read as unexpressive, angry, or depressed. In general, disability is relatively mild and lifespan is not affected.

■ Occurrence—It is an autosomal dominant disease, although it does appear sporadically with no family history of the disease. It affects both men and women in equal numbers and its prevalence is approximately 5 in 100,000 people.

■ Course—Symptoms usually are apparent between the first and third decades of life and are slowly progressive.

■ Pathology—Although the underlying genetic defect is not well understood, a deletion of a gene near the end of chromosome 4 has been identified in most people diagnosed with FSH. There are some indications that this genetic defect causes an over-expression of a specific protein (FRG1) that is linked to skeletal muscle defects and the health of retinal blood vessels.

■ Complications—In addition to weakness and loss of muscle tissue, patients may experience pain and inflammation in muscles and joints. Frozen joints and deformities caused by contractures are also possible. Progressive hearing loss in the

high frequencies is common and abnormalities of the retina are known to occur in FSH. Heart and lung involvement is rare.

■ Cognition—Mental retardation does occur in a subset of individuals with FSH, but is most likely to be found in those with large genetic deletions and early onset of muscle weakness.

■ Swallowing—Impairments in swallowing have been documented in close to 10% of patients with FSH. Involvement may include atrophy and weakness of the tongue, in addition to the impairment of lip function. Investigators have not identified involvement of pharyngeal or laryngeal muscles and functional affects appear to be limited to the oral stage of swallowing (Wohlgemuth et al., 2006).

6. Myotonic muscular dystrophy (MMD)
   ■ Overview—MMD is a relatively common form of MD that causes weakness and inability to relax muscles of the face, feet and hands. The term myotonia refers to an impaired ability to relax a muscle after it has been voluntarily contracted. In its mildest presentation, classified as Type 2 and sometimes referred to as proximal myotonic myopathia (PROMM), patients will develop muscle tone impairment and cataracts after the age of 20, with some not showing symptoms until the eighth decade of life. The more common Type 1 form of the disease (also known as Steinert's disease) accounts for 98% of cases and has two subtypes: a classical form and

congenital presentation. In the classical form, patients experience prominent myotonia and generalized muscle weakness and the disease is accompanied by hair loss, cataracts and heart rhythm disturbances. In these cases the symptoms are first detected between the ages of 10 to 30. The congenital form of Type 1 MMD is characterized by symptoms that are evident at birth. Infants have evidence of weakness, respiratory impairments and mental retardation.

■ Occurrence—This disease affects both men and women in about equal numbers. The congenital form of the disease occurs at a rate of about 1 in 100,000 births. Overall, MMD is found in about 1 in every 8,000 individuals.

■ Course—Depending on the type of myotonic dystrophy (mild, classical or congenital) symptoms may be evident any time from birth through geriatrics, with symptoms slowly progressing. The prognosis for the mild form is usually quite good with nonimpairing disabilities and a normal life expectancy. In the classical form of MMD the life span usually ranges from between 45 and 55 years and disability is more common. The congenital form is the most severe with respiratory and heart defects limiting life span to about 45 years.

■ Pathology—MMD is an inherited autosomal dominant pattern disease passed along to about 50% the offspring of carriers. The specific genetic defect differs for Type 1 and Type 2. In Type 1 the defect is known to be in a gene that codes for a protein essential for skeletal and cardiac muscle function, myotonic dystrophy protein kinase. For Type 2 disease the mutation occurs in a different gene with different proteins affected. Having a particular gene unit repeated too many times is the basic cause of myotonic dystrophies. They are considered to be "anticipation" diseases in that the offspring of a person with abnormally high repeat numbers will inherit even more repeats of the genetic unit. The result is that symptoms of the disease will tend to be more severe and appear at an earlier age than the parent.

■ Complications—MMD can affect different bodily tissues including the eyes, cardiac muscles, the endocrine system and the nervous system. In addition to the muscle weakness and myotonia, there can be respiratory impairments, deformities like clubfoot, smooth muscle impairments including the GI system, and developmental delays in cognitive, speech, language, and motor areas. Even in the milder forms of Type 2, cognitive and behavioral issues can be evident.

■ Cognition—There are variable degrees of cognitive impairment depending on the form of the disease. In the mild form, mental retardation is not evident. The classical presentation is marked by cognitive deficits across a range of impairments. In the congenital form of myotonic dystrophy there is more severe mental retardation that can severely limit independence.

- Swallowing—Swallowing problems are prevalent in all forms of myotonic dystrophy and can involve any or all stages of swallowing: oral, pharyngeal and esophageal. Later in this chapter the swallowing issues involved in myotonic dystrophy are described in detail.

7. Oculopharyngeal muscular dystrophy (OPMD)
   - Overview—OPMD is characterized by adult onset of weakness of the eyelids, causing ptosis, and the pharyngeal muscles, contributing to dysphagia. There are two forms of the disease: the much more common autosomal dominant type and extremely rare autosomal recessive form.
   - Occurrence—The disease is present in both men and women in approximately equal numbers. Overall the prevalence is estimated at 1 in 100,000 individuals; however, there are genetic clusters in which it appears much more commonly, that is, French-Canadian population of Quebec (1 in 1,000) and Bukharian Jews of Israel (1 in 600).
   - Course—The disease is slowly progressive beginning in adulthood. For the more common autosomal dominant form, the typical age for development of ptosis is about 48 (with a range of 26 to 65 years) and dysphagia appears at about 51 years of age (range 40 to 63) (Bouchard,

Brais, Brunet, Gould, & Roulea, 1997). The less common recessive form of OPMD tends to appear after the age of 60, with dysphagia symptoms developing after the age of 70.

- Pathology—The genetic defect appears to be in the PABPN1 protein (poly(A)-binding protein nuclear). Although the specific function of PABPN1 protein is unknown, it appears that the defective protein forms clumps, or intranuclear inclusions, to develop in muscles, thus impairing their function and eventually causing muscle cell death, or dystrophy. The reason for this to build up preferentially in ocular and pharyngeal muscles remains unknown.

- Complications—In addition to ptosis and dysphagia, proximal lower extremity weakness occurs in over 70% of individuals, with proximal upper extremity involvement found in about 40%. Other head and neck muscles are frequently impaired and include the vocal folds, tongue, face and extraocular muscles (Bouchard et al., 1997). Secondary complications associated with dysphagia are common and include aspiration pneumonia, weight loss, and social isolation related to embarrassment from choking. To compensate for ptosis, patients commonly tilt the neck backward, which in turn negatively impacts the cervical vertebrae and swallowing. Obstructive sleep apnea is also a potential problem related to weakness of musculature that supports the upper airway. Although OPMD does not generally reduce life span, quality of life is often impacted in later life (Becher et al., 2001).

- Cognition—Although cognitive decline is not generally associated with OPMD, there has been an identification of a subset of homozygote individuals (those inheriting the defective gene from each parent) who demonstrated a more severe form of the disease that included cognitive decline, recurrent depression and psychotic manifestations. These individuals developed symptoms by age 35 and died earlier, most in their 50s (Blumen et al., 2009).
- Swallowing—Typically, individuals with OPMD begin to have difficulties with solid food, manifested by increased time to complete a meal (Bouchard et al., 1997). As weakness progresses and begins to affect muscles beyond the pharyngeal constrictors, liquids can become problematic. Because dysphagia is a primary symptom of OPMD, this is discussed in detail later in this chapter.

8. Distal muscular dystrophy (DD)
- Overview—DD refers to a rare group of inherited muscular dystrophies in which the distal muscles of the hands and feet are most affected. Symptoms typically appear between the ages of 25 and 60, but juvenile forms of DD exist. In certain types of the disease other muscles may be affected in later life.
- Occurrence—The disease is considered to be very rare,

except in Sweden where it is more prevalent, with 8 cases per 100,000 individuals in certain regions (Westerberg, 1984).
- Course—The disease tends to be slowly progressive and nonlife-threatening.
- Pathology—DD may be either autosomal dominant or autosomal recessive. In the various forms of the disease, different proteins have been implicated. Dysferlin, a protein important in muscle repair, has been linked to DD.
- Complications—The degree of disability and affect on quality of life is dependent on the particular form of the disease and the physical demands of the individual.
- Cognition—Mental retardation and decline in cognitive function generally are not associated with DD.
- Swallowing—Typically the disease is confined to muscles of the arms and legs, but a "distal myopathy with vocal cord and pharyngeal weakness" has been reported and genetically mapped (Mastaglia & Laing, 1999). In these very rare cases, swallowing may be a feature.

9. Congenital muscular dystrophy (CMD)
- Overview—CMD refers to a class of muscular dystrophies in which symptoms are evident at or near birth.
- Occurrence—The frequency of CMD varies depending on the region in which it occurs and the form of the disease. For example, Fukuyama CMD is a relatively common form of the

disease found in Japan, with 7 to 12 cases per 100,000 children affected (Fukuyama, Kwazura, & Haruna, 1960). Forms of CMD occur at a rate of about 4 to 7 per 100,000 in various European countries.

- Course—Symptoms may be slowly progressive or non-progressive, with some forms shortening the life span.
- Pathology—CMDs are generally autosomal recessive, but can have a dominant pattern or occur sporadically because of a new genetic mutation. The disease may involve any number of proteins that can potentially affect the development of skeletal muscles, ocular muscles and the brain.
- Complications—Although some children progress from infancy into adulthood with minimal disability, others die very early from complications. Respiratory insufficiency, bulbar weakness, and seizures are possible in CMD. Joint contractures frequently are an issue that may need to be addressed by early therapeutic intervention.
- Cognition—Depending on the form of CMD, brain development can be impaired. For example, Fukuyama CMD involves mental retardation.
- Swallowing—One form of CMD, Walker-Warburg syndrome, presents with severe brain defects, hypotonia, and impaired sucking and swallowing. The average time to death in these infants is 9 months (Lopate, 2009). Abnormalities of the brain

and oral-pharyngeal structures are also evident in other forms of CMD.

Signs and Diagnostic Criteria

Because different types of MD affect different muscle groups, the signs and symptoms vary greatly from case to case. However, the following list generally is accepted as representative of the diagnostic criteria for MD:

- Delayed development of muscle skills and coordination
- Progressive muscle wasting
- Frequent falls
- Impaired gait (for example, waddling, walking on toes, poor balance) or inability to walk
- Calf pain and/or deformation, that is, enlargement
- Limited range of movement and joint contractures
- Scoliosis or curvature of the spine
- Respiratory impairments
- Ptosis
- Gonad atrophy
- Loss of bladder control
- Cataracts
- Frontal baldness
- Mental impairment

Many other symptoms may also be present in specific forms of MD. For example, myotonic muscles, dysphagia, gastrointestinal, and cardiac impairments are common for certain types of MD.

The diagnosis of MD is often difficult because of the heterogeneous symptoms and variable ages at which the impairments appear. In certain cases the risk for a child inheriting MD is known because of the parent history, but without this information diagnosis before age 2 or 3 is problematic and based on the child's achievement of developmental milestones and characteristic manner of walking, for example, waddling gait. Other causes, such as cerebral palsy, must be ruled out. As MD is genetic and usually inherited (although in rare instances new genetic mutations occur), family history is critical in the diagnostic process. Electromyography, ultrasonography, and muscle biopsy are common tests. Blood analysis to determine the level of creatine phosphokinase (CPK) is a critical test to determine the degree of muscle cell damage. A definitive diagnosis can be made on the basis of DNA analysis of blood.

Evolution

The evolution of MD is largely dependent on the form of inherited disease. However, cases within any of the nine categories of MD will vary according to the time of onset of symptoms and the degree of protein abnormality.

Epidemiology

The prevalence of MD, considered to be a rare disease, varies greatly depending on the type and the population in which it is measured. Duchenne muscular dystrophy, the most common, is diagnosed in 1 in every 3,600 males; whereas the congenital form myotonic dystrophy is found in only 1 in every 100,000 individuals. Certain genetically related groups of people are known to have much more common occurrences; for example, the oculopharyngeal form of the disease is found in 1 in every 600 Bukharian Jews in Israel.

Medical/Surgical Treatment

MD currently is an incurable disease. Current research in the area of gene therapy shows promise to perhaps stop the progression of certain forms of the disease (Chamberlain, 2002). Meanwhile, interventions are focused on symptomatic management to prevent or reduce the impact of disabling conditions. For example, deformities can be prevented or reduced in some by employing physical therapy, assistive devices, medications, and surgery. Physical therapists use range of motion exercises and targeted strengthening of specific muscles to maintain function. Braces and splints can be used to minimize contractures. Muscle spasms, stiffness and myotonia are affected by certain medications. Muscle deterioration is treated with anti-inflammatory corticosteroid medications and immunosuppressive drugs are prescribed to impede damage to muscle cells. When joint contractures are present, surgical tendon release procedures may be employed. Preventive measures, such as vaccinations for pneumonia and influenza, are also employed to avert complications from secondary infections.

It is important to recognize that impairments in swallowing are found in 7 of the 9 forms of MD described above. In the following sections, the swallowing impairments of MMD and OPMN are discussed in more detail.

Swallowing in Myotonic Muscular Dystrophy

Epidemiology

There has been a range of statistics reporting the prevalence of dysphagia in

MMD from 25 to 80% (Willig, Paulus, & Saint Guily, 1994). Ertekin, Yuceyar, Aydogdu, and Karasoy (2001) reported that there was objective evidence of dysphagia in approximately 70% of patients with MMD.

Pathology

It is clear that muscle impairments in MMD frequently contribute to swallowing difficulties. Even infants with congenital forms of this disease have been noted to have difficulties with sucking and swallowing. Feeding tubes are required for some to assure adequate nutrition during early life. When facial, lingual, and jaw weakness are evident, swallowing issues are likely to remain present throughout life.

As indicated above, MMD is a problem of muscle weakness and myotonia, or impaired ability to relax muscles that have been contracted. Weakness is a problem that is ubiquitous in muscular and neuromuscular diseases, but myotonia is a much less common phenomenon. The extent to which each contributes to the swallowing difficulties of patients with MMD has not been fully elucidated. The symptoms that define abnormal swallowing in this population can be largely explained on the basis of muscle weakness alone. For example, impaired chewing, nasal reflux, increased duration of swallowing phases, and even low upper esophageal sphincter pressure and reduced upper esophageal contractions can be attributed to reduced muscle strength. Using evidence from objective measures of swallowing, Leonard, Kendall, Johnson, and McKenzie (2001) concluded that it is weakness and not myotonia that accounts of the measurable changes in swallowing. However, based on the complaints from some of our patients of "cramping throat muscles" exacerbated by the ingestion of cold liquid and food, myotonia may be a contributing factor for at least some patients. In support of our observations, Ertekin and colleagues (2001) concluded that myotonia as well as weakness contributed to their findings of abnormal pharyngeal stage prolongations and should not be dismissed completely.

Adults with MMD may have impairments in any or all stages of swallowing. Relative to the oral stage, impaired chewing and bolus control have been reported (Odman & Kiliaridis, 1996) in patients with MMD. Drooling is associated with facial weakness and is common with congenital forms of MMD (Dodge, Gamstorp, Byers, & Russell, 1965). Nasal reflux was observed during videofluoroscopy in MMD patients who had early childhood or adolescent onset of disease (Hillarp, Ekberg, Jacobsson, Nylander, & Aberg, 1994).

Pharyngeal stage abnormalities have been measured and defined in terms of delays in triggering muscle contractions and prolongations of physiologic events. For example, delays in excitation of submental muscle contractions and prolonged laryngeal elevation have been measured (Ertekin et al., 2001). Functionally, choking appears to be one of the most common problems reported by patients with MMD (Willig et al., 1994). Pooling of saliva and residual material in the valleculae and piriform sinuses are commonly visualized during fluoroscopy and endoscopy procedures (Osanai, 2004). Leonard, Kendall, McKenzie, Gonsalves, and Walker (2000), using a novel approach for measuring the maximal pharyngeal area constricted during swallowing, described markedly reduced strength of pharyngeal contractions in MMD patients. Pharyngeal muscles may demonstrate asymmetric contractions as well.

At the level of the upper esophageal sphincter (UES), both manometric studies and electromyography have demonstrated abnormalities consisting of weak contractions and abnormal relaxation times (Modolell et al., 1999; Ertekin, 2001). With regard to the esophagus, patients with MMD demonstrate marked weakness of peristaltic contractions and delayed esophageal emptying (Eckardt, Nix, Kraus, & Bohl, 1986). Incomplete relaxation of the UES and hypotonia of the esophagus was reported as the most common abnormality detected on radiographic studies of swallowing (Marcon et al., 1998).

Clinical Intervention

It is not unusual for patients with MMD to ignore and even deny swallowing symptoms even when there are clear signs of impairment (Leonard, 2010). Given the insidious nature of the problem, the likelihood that patients have coped for many years with functional abnormalities and the possibility of cognitive deficits, it is not surprising that denial of impairment is common. Timely and appropriate intervention is dependent on careful assessment of any patient who is deemed at risk for complications brought on by swallowing dysfunction. Health care professionals should attend to signs of swallowing impairment such as weight loss, respiratory changes, and alterations in eating habits, diet, and time needed to complete a meal. Prompt referral to dysphagia specialists may obviate more severe complications.

Swallowing assessment for patients with MMD might include serial clinical examinations, a videofluoroscopic swallow study and videoendoscopic swallowing assessment. Since weak and myotonic muscles potentially impact all stages of swallowing, dynamic fluoroscopic swallow studies are particularly helpful in documenting the efficiency and effectiveness of all components of the deglutatory mechanism. MMD frequently impacts the oral-pharyngeal musculature by altering the timing needed for the sequential muscle contractions and releases that are required to swallow safely. Because of the prevalence of esophageal motility problems in MMD, barium esophagrams should be combined with the dynamic fluoroscopic swallow study.

Patient and caregiver education and counseling is an important aspect of intervention. Imaging studies can be particularly helpful in demonstrating for patients what is required to make swallowing more efficient and safe. Planned periodic follow-up usually is necessary to detect changes in function, determine the effectiveness of previous interventions and to help patients plan ahead. For some, planning may mean consideration of nonoral feeding routes.

Leonard (2010), in her chapter published in *Dysphagia in Rare Diseases*, describes a number of behavioral interventions that can be particularly helpful for patients with MMD. In particular she emphasizes that precautions be taken to avoid complications brought on by pharyngeal muscular weakness, gastroesophageal reflux, and impaired esophageal motility. For example, she recommends having the patient eat multiple small meals per day to counter the effects of fatigue. She reports that alternating thick and thin consistencies is helpful for some patients to reduce pharyngeal residue. The traditional strategies of head-turning and side-lying were not proven to be helpful in reducing pharyngeal pooling, even when there is demonstrated asymmetry in pharyngeal strength. In Leonard's experience, hard swallows and chin-down postures have been beneficial to some, but not all patients with MMD. Maneuvers like the supraglottic swallow and Mendelsohn that produce early and prolonged airway protection can also be beneficial when coughing, choking, and aspiration are an issue. Finally, because of the likelihood of esophageal abnormalities, she advocates that avoiding a supine position for at least 2 hours following a meal can help to prevent reflux aspiration.

Although the evidence is not clear regarding the relative contributions of weakness and myotonia to the swallowing impairments of patients with MMD, one should be cautious regarding the possible influence of cold on the pharyngeal and esophageal musculature. There is some evidence that cold can exacerbate muscular weakness in patients with MMD (Holmberg, Nordqvist, & Ahlström, 1996) and it is known that a cold stimulus can induce muscle spasms in the esophagus even for an unimpaired population (Meyer & Castell, 1981). Furthermore, although not well documented in MMD, certain forms of myotonia are made worse by a cold stimulus, for example in myotonia congenita and paramyotonia congenital, both rare inherited diseases caused by ion channel pathology. If the effect of cold on swallowing is a question that arises in a particular case, chilled barium can be used to study swallowing (Jones & Donner, 1988).

Swallowing in Oculopharyngeal Dystrophy

Epidemiology

Dysphagia, along with ptosis, is a cardinal symptom of OPMD. Objective evidence of abnormalities in the pharynx and/or esophagus is found in virtually all patients with this diagnosis (Castell, Castell, Duranceau, & Topart, 1995).

Pathology

OPMD is caused by muscle cell death and subsequent structural changes in musculature that is essential for normal swallowing. When biopsied, the cells are found to have deposits of intranuclear inclusions within the cells and the muscle tissue has excessive fatty replacement tissue. It is difficult to clinically detect atrophy because of the presence of fat versus muscle tissue, but there is microscopic evidence demonstrating that the atrophic changes of OPMD differ from neurogenic atrophy (Bouchard et al., 1997).

Functional abnormalities in swallowing have been reported in several facets of bolus transfer, transport and clearance. The changes are consistent with muscle weakness consistent with the loss of muscle fibers (Palmer, Neel, Sprouls, & Morrison, 2010). In evacuating a bolus from the oral cavity into the pharynx, there is a reduction in base of tongue to pharyngeal wall pressure (Palmer, 2010). Once the bolus enters the pharyngeal cavity, there is relatively high likelihood that nasal-pharyngeal reflux will occur on certain swallows (Périé et al., 1997). Measures of reduced pharyngeal pressures provide evidence for weakened constrictor musculature (Castell et al., 1995; Périé et al., 1997). At the level of the UES, there is abnormally timed and incomplete relaxation (Castell et al., 1995). Finally, the esophagus is also found to be abnormal in manometric studies of patients with OPMD. The esophageal anomalies were defined as dysmotility and incomplete lower esophageal sphincter relaxation (Castell et al., 1995).

Physiologic abnormalities contribute to major functional issues for patients with OPMD. The presence of pharyngeal residue often necessitates the patient to perform multiple swallows to clear a bolus; a maneuver that frequently is unsuccessful. Individuals may attempt to manage their difficulties by altering their diet, often eliminating certain foods and textures. Lengthening of the time required to eat a meal, weight loss, and malnutrition are complaints that can bring patients into the clinic for assessment of swallowing (de Swart et al., 2006). Other complications of dysphagia related to OPMD are aspiration pneumonia, possibly requiring intubation, prolonged hospitalization, and even death (Christopher, Horkan, Patterson, & Yodice, 2001; Périé et al., 1997).

Clinical Intervention

Patients with OPMD deserve a careful clinical assessment that includes a detailed history and inspection of oral-pharyngeal musculature. Videofluoroscopy and manometry of pharyngeal and esophageal musculature are the most valuable techniques for instrumentally evaluating swallowing in patients with OPMD (Palmer, 2010). Describing the specific abnormalities in the swallowing musculature is critically important to the employment of effective compensatory behaviors and maneuvers.

Muscle strengthening exercises designed to improve swallowing and focused on oral-pharyngeal musculature for patients with OPMD are of questionable benefit. Endurance and aerobic training have been shown to benefit patients with BMD and FSH, but these exercises were directed toward measures of fitness, such as maximal oxygen uptake (Olsen, Orngreen, & Vissing, 2005) and large muscle strength, specifically leg extension (Sveen et al., 2008). In a study of a small number of OPMD patients, Zochodne and colleagues (1992) found that submaximal strengthening exercises of the forearm flexor muscles resulted in an increase of exercise-induced acidosis and muscles recovered more slowly as compared to control subjects. The implication is that OPMD subjects demonstrate an abnormal metabolic response to exercise compared to normal subjects. Palmer (2010) has observed improved swallowing function in patients with OPMD, specifically increased intraoral pressure generation, following submaximal "warm-up" type exercises. Furthermore, it was noted that patients benefited from stretching and range of motion exercises to reduce muscle stiffness. Taken as a whole, therefore, the most prudent approach to the employment of exercises for patients with OPMD is to avoid those that focus on increasing maximal strength by fatiguing muscles and direct exercises to those that maintain range of motion and "warm-up" muscles through more gentle stretching.

Special attention should be paid to the neck posture of patients with OPMD during swallowing. Because of bilateral ptosis, individuals frequently will retroflex their neck in order to see. This neck extension posture with the head tilted back has a negative impact on swallowing. Investigators have demonstrated that by adjusting the posture of OPMD patients to a slightly neck flexed position, both subjective and objective measures of function were improved (deSwart et al., 2006).

Nasal-pharyngeal reflux (NPR) presents a problem for many patients with OPMD. Some clinicians have advocated for the fitting of a palatal lift prostheses to help control for NPR (Palmer, 2010). Most of the benefits from the prosthesis may occur for non-deglutatory functions, that is, decreasing hypernasality in speech. Some patients may not be able to swallow effectively with the prosthesis in place.

A common and prominent feature of the dysphagia associated with OPMD is UES dysfunction. Ill-timed relaxation and incomplete opening of this sphincter contribute to the functional impairment. Approaches to treating this problem have included dilation, botulinum toxin (BOTOX®) injection, and myotomy. Dilation of the UES has reportedly brought relief of symptoms for about 65% of OPMD patients, with benefits lasting for up to 18 months in some cases (Mathieu et al., 1997). Specific outcome data following BOTOX® injections of the UES have not been reported for this population, however, some benefits have been described as occurring within two weeks of injection (Marchese-Ragona, Marioni, Restivo, & Staffieri, 2005). The surgical approach, cricopharyngeal myotomy, has been found to have longer term benefits for some OPMD patients. Coiffier, Périé, Laforet, Eymard, and St. Guily (2006) reported that 90% of their 39 patients who underwent myotomy had positive benefits with 25 showing complete remission of dysphagia symptoms. These investigators and others have pointed out that even with successful cricopharyngeal myotomy procedures, dysphagia symptoms commonly reappear gradually over the ensuing years (Duranceau, 1997).

Behavioral adjustments to diet are beneficial. Palmer (2010) recommends for some patients to alternate between liquid and solid boluses or perform multiple swallows per bolus to reduce pharyngeal residue. Because for many patients meals take longer and this can lead to problems of weight loss and malnutrition, diets that are calorie dense and highly nutritious can help to obviate these issues. Mealtime logs can help dietitians in adjusting diets and identifying bolus textures that potentially are dangerous.

SUMMARY

Myopathies, as opposed to neuropathies and neuronal pathway diseases, are due to a defect at the level of muscle fibers. Because the clinical manifestation of the myopathies overlaps with disorders of the peripheral and central nervous systems, and because peripheral neural fibers often show signs of secondary pathology, they commonly are described as neuromuscular impairments. Dysphagia is a problem found commonly in individuals with inflammatory myopathies (for example, inclusion body myositis, polymyositis and dermatomyositis), and it is highly prevalent in certain forms of MD, a hereditary etiology for myopathy. For individuals diagnosed with MMD and OPMD, dysphagia symptoms are described in all stages of swallowing. Those with MMD may have difficulties associated with weakness of muscle contractions, as well as problems relaxing muscles following contraction—myotonia. Effective intervention centers on the need for careful assessment, including the possibility that certain sensory properties, for example cold, may elicit overly strong muscle contractions and exacerbate difficulties relaxing muscles during a swallow. Dysphagia described in patients with OPMD is associated with an inability to generate adequate muscle force and affects all phases of swallowing extending from oral clearance to lower esophageal sphincter relaxation. Interventions are focused on the management of specific symptoms, for example, nasal regurgitation, and the institution of submaximal "warm-up" and stretching exercises.

REFERENCES

Aloysius, A., Born, P., Kinali, M., Davis, T., Pane, M., & Mercuri E. (2008). Swallowing difficulties in Duchenne muscular dystrophy: Indications for feeding assessment and outcome of videofluroscopic swallow studies. *European Journal of Paediatric Neurology, 12*, 239-245.

Angelini, C., Fanin, M., Pegoraro, E. Freda, M. P., Cadaldini, M., & Martinello, F. (1994). Clinical-molecular correlation in 104 mild X-linked muscular dystrophy patients: Characterization of sub-clinical phenotypes. *Neuromuscular Disorders, 4*, 349-358.

Becher, M. W., Morrison, L., Davis, L. E., Maki, W. C., King, M. K., Bicknell, J. M., . . . Bear, D. G.. (2001). Oculopharyngeal muscular dystrophy in Hispanic New Mexicans. *Journal of the American Medical Association, 286*, 2437-2440.

Blumen, S. C., Bouchard, J. P., Brais, B., Carasso R. L., Paleacu, D., V. Droryet, V. E., . . . Braverman, I. (2009). Cognitive impairment and reduced life span of oculopharyngeal muscular dystrophy homozygotes. *Neurology, 73*, 596-601.

Bouchard, J. P., Brais, B., Brunet, D., Gould, P. V., & Roulea, G. A. (1997). Recent studies on oculopharyngeal muscular dystrophy in Québec. *Neuromuscular Disorders, 7*, S22-S29.

Castell, J. A., Castell, D. O., Duranceau, A., & Topart, P. (1995). Manometric characteristics of the pharynx, upper esophageal sphincter, esophagus, and lower esophageal sphincter in patients with oculopha-

ryngeal muscular dystrophy. *Dysphagia, 10*, 22-26.

Chamberlain, J. S. (2002). Gene therapy of muscular dystrophy. *Human Molecular Genetics, 11*, 2355-2362.

Christopher, K., Horkan, C., Patterson, R. B., & Yodice, P. C. (2001). Oculopharyngeal muscular dystrophy complicating airway management. *Chest, 120*, 2101-2103.

Coiffier, L., Périé, S., Laforet, P., Eymard, B., & St Guily, J. L. (2006). Long-term results of cricopharyngeal myotomy in oculopharyngeal muscular dystrophy. *Otolaryngology-Head and Neck Surgery, 135*, 218-222.

Dalakas, M., & Hohlfeld, R. (2003). Polymyositis and dermatomyositis. *Lancet, 362*(9388), 971-982.

deSwart, B. J. M., van der Sluijs, B. M., Vos, A. M. C., Kalf, J. G., Knuijt, S., Cruysberg, J. R. M., & van Engelen, B. G. M. (2006). Ptosis aggravates dysphagia in oculopharyngeal muscular dystrophy. *Journal of Neurology, Neurosurgery and Psychiatry, 77*, 266-268.

Dodge, P. R., Gamstorp, I., Byers, R. K., & Russell, P. (1965). Myotonic dystrophy in infancy and childhood. *Pediatrics, 35*, 3-19.

Duranceau, A. (1997). Cricopharyngeal myotomy in the management of neurogenic and muscular dysphagia. *Neuromuscular Disorders, 7*, S85-S89.

Eckardt, V. F., Nix, W., Kraus, W., & Bohl, J. (1986). Esophageal motor function in patients with muscular dystrophy. *Gastroenterology, 90*, 628-635.

Ertekin, C., Yuceyar, N., Aydogdu, I., & Karasoy, H. (2001). Electrophysiological evaluation of oropharyngeal swallowing in myotonic dystrophy. *Journal of Neurology, Neurosurgery and Psychiatry, 70*, 363-371.

Fukuyama, Y., Kwazura, M., & Haruna, H. (1960). A peculiar form of congenital muscular dystrophy. *Paediatric University of Tokyo, 4*, 5-8.

Giliberto, F., Ferreiro, V., Dalamon, V., & Szijan, I. (2004). Dystrophin deletions and cognitive impairment in Duchenne/Becker muscular dystrophy. *Neurological Research,* *26,* 83–87.

Hanayama, K., Liu, M., Higuchi, Y., Fujiwara, T., Tsuji, T., Hase, K., & Ishihara, T. (2008). Dysphagia in patients with Duchenne muscular dystrophy evaluated with a questionnaire and videofluorography. *Disability Rehabilitation, 30,* 517–522.

Hillarp, B., Ekberg, O., Jacobsson, S., Nylander, G., & Aberg, M. (1994) Myotonic dystrophy revealed at videoradiography of deglutition and speech in adult patients with velopharyngeal insufficiency: Presentation of four cases. *Cleft Palate-Craniofacial Journal, 31,* 125–133.

Hinton, V. J., De Vivo, D. C., Nereo, N. E., Goldstein, E., & Stern, Y. (2000). Poor verbal working memory across intellectual level in boys with Duchenne dystrophy. *Neurology, 54,* 2127–2132.

Holmberg, E., Nordqvist, K., & Ahlström, G. (1996). Prevalence of dysarthria in adult myotonic dystrophy (M. Steinert) patients: Speech characteristics and intelligibility. *Logopedics Phoniatrics Vocology, 21,* 21–27.

Houser, S. M., Calabrese, L. H., & Strome, M. (1998). Dysphagia in patients with inclusion body myositis. *Laryngoscope, 108*(7), 1001–1005.

Jones, B., & Donner, M. W. (1988). Examination of the patient with dysphagia. *Radiology, 167,* 319–326.

Leonard, R. J. (2010). Myotonic muscular dystrophy (MMD). In H. Jones, & J. Rosenbek (Eds.), *Dysphagia in rare conditions* (pp. 401–408). San Diego, CA: Plural.

Leonard, R. J., Kendall, K. A., Johnson, R., & McKenzie, S. (2001). Swallowing in myotonic muscular dystrophy: A videofluoroscopic study. *Archives of Physical Medicine and Rehabilitation, 82,* 979–985.

Leonard, R. J., Kendall, K. A., McKenzie, S., Gonsalves, M. I., & Walker, A. (2000). Structural displacements in normal swallowing: A videofluoroscopic study. *Dysphagia, 15,* 146–152.

Lopate, G. (2009). Congenital muscular dystrophy. eMedicine. Retrieved February 12, 2009, from: http://emedicine.medscape .com/article/1180214-overview

Marchese-Ragona, R., Marioni, G., Restivo, D. A., & Staffieri, A. (2005). Solving dysphagia due to cricopharyngeal muscle dysfunction with botulinum toxin. *European Archives of Oto-Rhino-Laryngology, 262,* 250–251.

Marcon, M., Briani, C., Ermani, M., Menegazzo, E., Iurilli ,V., Feltrin, G. P., . . . Angelini, C. (1998). Positive correlation of CTG expansion and pharyngoesophageal alterations in myotonic dystrophy patients. *Italian Journal of Neurological Science, 19,* 75–80.

Mastaglia, F. L., & Laing, N. G. (1999). Distal myopathies: clinical and molecular diagnosis and classification. *Journal of Neurology, Neurosurgery and Psychiatry, 67,* 703–707.

Mathieu, J., Lapointe, G., Brassard, A., Tremblay, C., Brais, B., Rouleau, G. A., & Bouchard, J-P. (1997). A pilot study on upper esophageal sphincter dilation for the treatment of dysphagia in patients with oculopharyngeal muscular dystrophy. *Neuromuscular Disorders, 7,* 100–104.

Meyer, G. W., & Castell, D. O. (1981). Human esophageal response during chest pain induced by swallowing cold liquids. *Journal of the American Medical Association, 246,* 2057–2059.

Modolell, I., Mearin, F., Baudet, J. S., Gamez, J., Cervera, C., & Malagelada, J. R. (1999). Pharyngo-esophageal motility disturbances in patients with myotonic dystrophy. *Scandinavian Journal of Gastroenterology, 34,* 878–882.

Nozaki, S., Umaki, Y., Sugishita, S., Tatara, K., Adachi, K., & Shinno S. (2007). Videofluorographic assessment of swallowing function in patients with Duchenne muscular dystrophy. *Rinsho Shinkeigaku, 47,* 407–412.

Odman, C. & Kiliaridis, S. (1996). Masticatory muscle activity in myotonic dystrophy patients. *Journal of Oral Rehabilitation, 23,* 5–10.

Oh, T. H., Brumfield, K. A., Hoskin, T. L., Kasperbauer, J. L., & Basford, J. R. (2008). Dysphagia in inclusion body myositis:

Clinical features, management, and clinical outcome. *American Journal of Physical Medicine and Rehabilitation, 87*, 883–889.

Olsen, D. B., Orngreen, M. C., & Vissing, J. (2005) Aerobic training improves exercise performance in facioscapulohumeral muscular dystrophy. *Neurology, 64*, 1064–1066.

Osanai, R. (2004). Swallowing disorder in patients with myotonic dystrophy type I. *Otolaryngology-Head and Neck Surgery, 131*, 284.

Palmer, P. M. (2010). Oculopharyngeal muscular dystrophy (OPMD). In H. Jones & J. Rosenbek (Eds.), *Dysphagia in rare conditions* (pp. 431–441). San Diego, CA: Plural.

Palmer, P. M., Neel, A. T., Sprouls, G., & Morrison, L. (2010). Swallow characteristics in patients with oculopharyngeal muscular dystrophy. *Journal of Speech, Language, and Hearing Research, 53*, 1567–1578.

Pane, M., Vasta, I., Messina, S., Sorleti, D., Aloysius, A., Sciarra F, . . . Mercuri, E. (2006). Feeding problems and weight gain in Duchenne muscular dystrophy. *European Journal of Paediatric Neurology, 10*, 231–236.

Périé, S., Eymard, B., Laccourreye, L., Chaussade, S., Fardeau, M., & St. Guily, J. L. (1997). Dysphagia in oculopharyngeal muscular dystrophy: A series of 22 French cases. *Neuromuscular Disorders, 7*, S96–S99.

Quijano-Roy, S., Renault, F., Romero, N., Guicheney, P., Fardeau, M., & Estournet B. (2004). EMG and nerve conduction studies in children with congenital muscular dystrophy. *Muscle and Nerve, 29*, 292–299.

Sveen, M. L., Jeppesen, T. D., Hauerslev, S., Køber, L., Krag, T. O., & Vissing, J. (2008).

Endurance training improves fitness and strength in patients with Becker muscular dystrophy. *Brain, 131*, 2824–2831.

Terzi, N., Prigent, H., Lejaille, M., Falaize, L., Annane, D., Orlikowski, D., & Lovaso, F. (2010). Impact of tracheostomy on swallowing performance in Duchenne muscular dystrophy. *Neuromuscular Disorders, 20*, 493–498.

Westerberg, B. (1984). Neuropediatric aspects of hereditary peripheral neuropathies in childhood. *International Journal of Rehabilitation Research, 7*, 65–67.

Willig, T. N., Paulus, J., & Saint Guily, J. L. (1994). Swallowing problems in neuromuscular disorders. *Archives of Physical Medicine and Rehabilitation, 75*, 1175–1181.

Wintzen, A. R., Bots, G. T., de Bakker, H. M., Hulshof, J. H., & Padberg, G. W. (1988). Dysphagia in inclusion body myositis. *Journal of Neurology, Neurosurgery and Psychiatry, 51*, 1542–1545.

Wohlgemuth, M., de Swart, B. J. M., Kalf, J. G., Joosten, A. M., Van der Vliet & Padberg, G. W. (2006). Dysphagia in facioscapulohumeral muscular dystrophy. *Neurology, 66*, 1926–1928.

Yu, W-M, Yu, H., & Chen, Z-L. (2007). Laminins in peripheral nerve development and muscular dystrophy. *Molecular Neurobiology, 35*, 288–297.

Zochodne, D. W., Koopman, W. J., Thompson, T., Driedger, A. A., Gravelle, D., & Bolton, C. F. (1992). Forearm P-31 nuclear magnetic resonance spectroscopy studies in oculopharyngeal muscular dystrophy. *Canadian Journal of Neurological Sciences, 19*, 174–179.

9 Neuromuscular Junction Disease

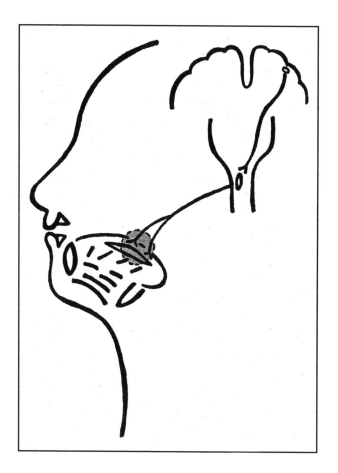

NEUROMUSCULAR JUNCTION

A neuromuscular junction (NMJ) is a physical intersection that exists between an axon in the peripheral nervous system and a muscle fiber. Functionally, the NMJ is a synapse that allows for the transmission of an action potential from an axon terminal of a motor neuron to a motor end plate, the excitable region of a muscle fiber's surface. In order for a signal to pass across the NMJ and trigger a contraction of the corresponding muscle fiber, the neurotransmitter acetylcholine (ACh) is released from the axon terminal into the synaptic cleft and binds to receptors located on the muscle fiber. The chemically induced change of an action potential at the motor end plate, referred to as end plate potential (EEP), generates a muscle fiber contraction (Figure 9–1). To terminate the action of ACh on the postsynaptic membrane, the degrading chemical enzyme acetylcholinesterase (AChE) is released into the synaptic cleft.

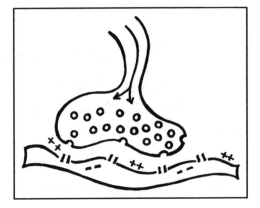

Figure 9–1. Neuromuscular junction. An impulse traveling down the length of an axon reaches the axon terminal to trigger the release of acetylcholine (ACh) into the synaptic cleft, the space formed between the axon membrane and muscle fiber. ACh molecules bind to receptors located along the length of muscle fibers to induce action potentials that in turn induce the fibers to contract.

NMJ DISEASES AND SYNDROMES

The multistep process of neural transmission at the NMJ can be impaired at any of several points. Most commonly, the EPP fails to activate effective and efficient muscle contractions because the ACh receptors have been disrupted by disease, as is the case with myasthenia gravis (MG). However, failure of a muscle fiber to contract may also result from a malfunction in the release of ACh from the presynaptic membrane. For example, the release of ACh is triggered by the uptake of calcium ions into the axon terminal. When voltage-gated calcium channels on the presynaptic membrane are blocked, calcium ions cannot enter and ACh cannot be released into the synaptic cleft. This condition is found in the condition Lambert-Eaton myasthenic syndrome (LEMG). ACh release also can be blocked by the effect of various toxins, for example, botulism. In this chapter we focus our attention on MG, the most common disease of the NMJ, and briefly describe LEMG with its contrasting

symptoms. In addition to MG and LEMG, a categorization of diseases and conditions that disrupt neural transmission at the NMJ includes:

- Congenital, familial myasthenia
- NMJ blockers (curare, botulism)
- Drug-induced myasthenic syndromes
- Tetanus

MYASTHENIA GRAVIS

Definition

Myasthenia gravis (MG) is considered to be in the class of autoimmune disorders and is a neuromuscular disease with impairment at the level of the neuromuscular junction (NMJ). It affects voluntary, skeletal muscles causing a progressive reduction in muscle strength with repeated use. After a period of rest, muscle strength recovers. The name is derived from Latin and Greek origins and literally means "grave muscle weakness." In MG the body's immune system produces antibodies that destroy, block, or disrupt the function of ACh receptors at the NMJ, thus interfering with repeated muscle contractions. Bulbar muscles, those innervated by cranial nerves, commonly are involved and include muscles that maintain eyelid opening, maintain jaw closure, and those that contract during speech and swallowing. Spinal muscles of the arms and, less commonly, the legs may be involved. Even the muscles of breathing can become too weak to support respiration, leading to a myasthenic crisis. As the pathology is at the NMJ, sensory functions remain intact; however, because of disturbances in muscles around the eyes, associated visual problems are common.

MG occurs more frequently in families with a history of autoimmune diseases and particularly in people who have more than one autoimmune disease. Coexisting thyroid disease, for example, is not uncommon.

An inherited form of MG exists that is caused by a genetic defect, and there is a transient neonatal condition that can occur in infants born to mothers with MG, presumably caused by the transfer of the mother's antibodies to the infant. In adult onset MG, a defect in the function of the thymus gland is frequently implicated. This small gland located beneath the sternum is part of the body's immune system and in MG it is thought to produce the antibodies that attack certain ACh receptors. Up to 75% of patients diagnosed with MG have identifiable abnormalities of the thymus, with the presence of a thymoma, or tumor on the gland, evident in 25% of patients.

Signs and Diagnostic Criteria

Many of the symptoms of MG are found in other diseases and conditions, thus making diagnosis challenging. Commonly, drooping eyelids and double vision, either horizontal or vertical, will be initial complaints. Impaired chewing and swallowing also are common presenting problems, although some patients will present with generalized fatigue. The typical complaint also will specify that weakness worsens as muscles are used repeatedly and/or symptoms will tend to increase toward the end of the day. With regard to speech, increased nasality might be evident after talking continuously for a few minutes. Chewing and swallowing worsens throughout a meal and is evident when food requires extensive chewing, like steak. Interestingly, those muscles that must function by sustaining contractions to lift structures against gravity are most susceptible to myasthenic fatigue. For example, the muscles of the eyelids sustain contractions to keep the eyes open during waking hours (Figure 9–2); the jaw muscles contract continuously to keep the jaw closed; and during speech, the velum remains elevated against gravity throughout most of a discourse.

Weijnen and associates (2000) report measurable decreases in lateral tongue force for patients with MG. Tongue atrophy also has been reported in rare instances and may be accompanied by atrophy of the velar muscles (Burch et al, 2006; De Assis et al, 1994).

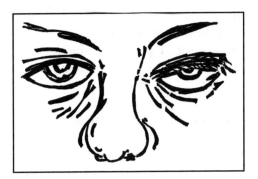

Figure 9–2. Bilateral ptosis of the upper eyelids. Muscles that must sustain contraction to work continuously against gravity, for example, the eyelids, are susceptible to fatigue and drooping when ACh is depleted, as is common in MG.

Neurologic examination of patients with MG typically will demonstrate normal reflexes and sensory testing. The motor tests may bring out a patient's ptosis of the eyelids by having the individual look upward for 30 seconds. Other techniques to stress the musculature and bring out muscle fatigue include keeping the arms outstretched for a minute, walking on the heels and then toes, and attempting to maintain arm and leg posture against resistance. Other diagnostic tests fall into the following categories: blood analysis, edrophonium test, imaging, and neurophysiology testing.

■ *Blood analysis* is used to detect abnormally elevated serum antibodies to the ACh receptors.

■ The *edrophonium test*, also known as a Tensilon test, involves intravenous administration of this drug, an ACh inhibitor, that blocks the breakdown of ACh and rapidly, although temporarily, increases the level of ACh available at NMJs. Once injected, patients with MG experience a brief period of im-

proved muscle strength; for example, drooping of eyelids will improve and speech that was hypernasal will improve, sometimes dramatically.

■ *Imaging*, including chest x-ray, computed tomography (CT), or magnetic resonance imaging (MRI) is used to identify abnormalities of the thymus gland or a thymoma.

■ *Neurophysiology tests* include nerve conduction studies, repetitive nerve stimulation, and single fiber electromyography (EMG). Nerve conduction studies involve the application of an electrical stimulus to an area of skin overlying a nerve and measuring the time it takes for the stimulus to trigger a muscle response. Electrodes placed at the point of electrical stimulation and on the skin over the muscle allow for a recording of rate of nerve conduction and the degree of muscle response. In repetitive nerve stimulation, the nerve is repeatedly stimulated and the fatigability of the muscle measured. Single fiber EMG, considered the most sensitive test for MG, requires insertion of a thin needle electrode into a muscle and recording potentials from individual muscle fibers. Specifically, examiners find two muscle fibers supplied by the same motor unit and measure the jitter, or variability in the firing patterns.

The Myasthenia Gravis Foundation of America has proposed a classification system based on which skeletal muscles are affected. It includes the following five classes:

■ Class I: Any eye muscle weakness, possible ptosis, no other evidence of muscle weakness elsewhere

- Class II: Eye muscle weakness of any severity, mild weakness of other muscles
  - Class IIa: Predominantly limb or axial muscles
  - Class IIb: Predominantly bulbar and/or respiratory muscles
- Class III: Eye muscle weakness of any severity, moderate weakness of other muscles
  - Class IIIa: Predominantly limb or axial muscles
  - Class IIIb: Predominantly bulbar and/or respiratory muscles
- Class IV: Eye muscle weakness of any severity, severe weakness of other muscles
  - Class IVa: Predominantly limb or axial muscles
  - Class IVb: Predominantly bulbar and/or respiratory muscles (Can also include feeding tube without airway intubation)
- Class V: Intubation needed to maintain airway

Evolution

The presentation and progression of MG are variable. In a large study of over 1,000 patients, between the years 1940 and 1980, the following initial symptoms were reported: ptosis 25%, diplopia 25%, blurred vision 3%, leg weakness 13%, generalized fatigue 6%, dysphagia 6%, and dysarthria 5% (Grob et al., 1981). Muscle atrophy can be found in a small percentage of patients with MG, even in the facial and lingual muscles (Oosterhuis, 1989). From initial onset a patient might progress from mild forms of the disease to a more severe condition over several weeks to months. Although it might remain isolated to the ocular muscles for years and

progression is not inevitable, when it does spread it typically moves from eye muscles to facial and other bulbar muscles and then to the trunk and limbs. In 16% of patients the disease remains isolated to ocular muscles and 87% progress to more generalized forms of the disease within 13 months of onset. Complete and spontaneous remission is extremely rare. The rate of mortality is presently 3 to 4%, with risk factors being over 40 years of age, a short course of severe symptoms, and the presence of a thymoma.

Epidemiology

The MG Foundation of America puts the prevalence of cases in the United States at 14 to 20 per 100,000 population. Therefore, there are between 36,000 and 60,000 persons with MG in the United States at any given time. The disease can occur at any age, but is most common in women and typically develops in the second and third decades of life. For men the onset is usually after the age of 50. A familial predisposition to MG is present in about 5% of cases.

Medical/Surgical Treatment

Patients with MG tend to respond favorably to treatment. One of the first lines of treatment is the administration of a chemical that inhibits the enzyme cholinesterase and prevents it from breaking down ACh. The administration of an acetylcholinesterase inhibitor drug, such as neostigmine (brand names: Prostigmin and Vagostigmin) or pyridostigmine (brand name: Mestinon), increases the amount of ACh and the duration that it is available to produce muscle contractions.

A second line of medication treatment utilizes immunosuppressive drugs (for example, prednisone, a corticosteroid; cyclosporine and azathioprine) to reduce the body's ability to produce ACh receptor antibodies. They are prescribed frequently for patients who have not responded fully to anticholinesterase drugs. These drugs are used with close monitoring as they may cause major side effects.

When a rapid response is required, as when patients face life-threatening situations like impending respiratory failure or severe dysphagia, high dose immune globulin therapy or plasma exchange may be utilized. In these therapies, the body's immune system is temporarily altered by the introduction of normal antibodies from donated blood. Another potential therapy is plasmapheresis, a process whereby the fluid component of a patient's blood, the plasma, is separated from the cells by processes of either high-speed spinning of the blood or filtering through a fine permeable membrane. Once separated, the blood cells are returned to the patient along with other fluids, while the plasma containing the abnormal antibodies is discarded.

Surgical removal of the thymus gland, thymectomy, is a relatively frequent procedure for patients with MG. The procedure is based on the fact that the thymus gland has been implicated as a component of the body's immune system, and extensive evidence from animal models suggests that impairment in the gland contributes to the development of MG. Although the surgery is indicated for the 10 to 15% of patients with evidence of thymoma, removal of the thymus remains somewhat controversial for others. Lymphoid follicular hyperplasia is found to be present in about 70% of cases, but the evidence for benefits of thymectomy for these individuals is not strong. Additionally, the timing of the surgery remains an issue (Bril & Keshavjee, 2007).

Patients with MG almost always have to make adjustments in lifestyle. Avoidance of stress and heat exposure are important as both can exacerbate symptoms. Activities are planned and adjusted to allow for scheduled rest periods. Determinations can be made regarding peak energy levels corresponding to medication affects, and activities planned around these times. Safety precautions and adaptations frequently are recommended for the home; for example, grab bars, railings, and nonslip mats can be beneficial. Measures are taken to avoid having eyes dry out when lid closure is incomplete, and eye patches are worn to help alleviate double vision.

Swallowing in Myasthenia Gravis

Epidemiology

Impairments in oropharyngeal musculature have been reported as a presenting symptom in 30% of patients with MG (Beekman, Kuks, & Oosterhuis, 1997; Salazar et al., 2002). Most investigators report that dysphagia and respiratory impairment are significant sources for both morbidity and mortality in MG. Ertekin, Yuceyar, and Aydogduand (1998) report that submental and laryngeal elevator muscles are demonstrated to respond abnormally on electrophysiologic studies, even in the absence of clinical signs of dysphagia. Specifically, they reported that submental muscles were activated for an abnormally long period of time during swallowing, thus laryngeal elevation was prolonged. This evidence for a subclinical impairment suggests that a higher number of patients with MG may be susceptible to swallowing difficulties and consequent complications when they become decompensated by illness, stress, or other exacerbating factors.

Physiology

There is a scarcity of studies describing the characteristics of swallowing in patients with MG. This partially can be explained on the basis of the variability in presentation of the disease, the fact that most patients respond to the medical management provided, and observations that each patient's symptoms vary depending on factors related to fatigue and timing of medication. Colton-Hudson et al. (2002) identified 20 patients with MG, all of whom described some degree of swallowing difficulty, and administered clinical and videofluoroscopic swallowing assessments. With regard to each stage of oropharyngeal swallowing, the investigators described the following:

■ Oral-preparatory: poor bolus formation with tongue (7/20); extended chewing, reduced buccal muscle tone and loss of material in lateral sulci (2/20)
■ Oral: slow transport (13/20); piecemeal deglutition (13/20); residue on base of tongue and soft palate (16/20); poor seal of soft palate to posterior tongue (15/20)
■ Pharyngeal: delayed initiation (20/20); reduced tongue base retraction (17/20); reduced epiglottic motility (12/20); residue in valleculae (17/20); residue in piriform sinuses (14/20).

The investigators also described laryngeal penetration with at least one bolus consistency in 13 of the 20 patients. Aspiration below the vocal folds occurred in 7 of 20 patients, 4 of whom did so silently. Interestingly, all 20 subjects in this study had at least mild flaccid dysarthria that typically was characterized by hypernasality (13/20), breathy or hoarse dysphonia (19/20), and imprecise articulation (13/20).

Aspiration appears to occur in an alarming percentage of patients with MG who experience swallowing difficulty (Koopman et al., 2004). Higo and colleagues (2005) performed 23 videofluoroscopic studies on 11 patients who were referred for swallowing assessment. They detected aspiration in almost 35% of cases and half of these occurred silently. Three of the four patients with silent aspiration went on to develop aspiration pneumonia. Analysis of their findings indicates that impaired laryngeal elevation significantly correlated with aspiration, and incomplete upper esophageal sphincter (UES) opening was a common finding.

The findings reported above supported earlier observations of Kluin and associates (1996). Reporting on 8 elderly patients with MG, they noted "fatigable flaccid dysarthria" in all patients. Additionally, all had decreased pharyngeal motility with residue in the valleculae and pyriform sinuses postswallowing; 5 of the 8 had UES impressions on fluoroscopic examinations; and 7 patients demonstrated aspiration, 5 silently. Ertekin and colleagues (1998) reported on 15 patients with swallowing impairments related to MG. Although they found no impairments in the CP sphincter per se, they indicated that function may be disturbed due to problems coordinating laryngeal elevation with sphincter relaxation. Their electrophysiologic measures also detected that during dry and wet swallowing patients with MG and dysphagia held their larynx in its elevated position for significantly longer than either age-matched controls or patients with MG without dysphagia.

Medications used to treat MG appear to have a positive effect on swallowing. In their electrophysiologic assessment of 15 patients with MG and dysphagia, Ertekin and colleagues (1998) described a range of severity: from patients who required a feeding tube to those with minor symptoms. In all instances anticholinesterase and corticosteroid treatment resulted in "appreciable recovery from dysphagia" (Ertekin et al., 1998). Using intraluminal pressure recordings and rapid serial radiography, Kramer and associates (1957) assessed 2 patients with MG immediately before and 20 minutes after administration of prostigmin. They report modest increases in intrapharyngeal pressures after taking the medication. These findings are consistent with earlier reports from Schwab and Viets (1941) in which they reported radiographic evidence of reduced pharyngeal residue in 17 of 20 patients after administration of prostigmin. The only contradictory report comes from Kluin and colleagues (1996) in which they studied elderly patients with MG and dysphagia and noted that although anticholinesterase and corticosteroid drugs improved the clinical course for these patients, there were no significant changes in measurable pharyngeal stage swallowing abnormalities.

In a study of 25 patients with MG, Huang and colleagues (1988) performed esophageal manometry and compared results to 20 normal control subjects. Ninety-six percent of the MG patients demonstrated abnormal motility, but no significant lower esophageal sphincter dysfunc-tion. In describing esophageal function, the investigators reported de-creased amplitude and prolongation of peristaltic waves. Furthermore, they noted a significant decrease in the upper esophageal sphincter pressure. Llabres and associates (2005) confirmed these findings in 2 subjects by showing generalized weakness of peristalsis, including the smooth segment of the esophagus. They reported that the impairment worsened with repeated swallows. Linke et al. (2003) also reported impairments in esophageal motility and transit time using noninvasive scintigraphy and recommended this as a method of routinely assessing esophageal function in patients with confirmed MG.

The effect of MG on respiratory muscles, particularly the diaphragm and thoracic chest wall muscles, may be manifested by a shallow tidal breathing pattern (Keenan et al., 1995; Garcia Rio et al., 1994) and reduced respiratory endurance (Heliopoulos et al., 2003). Commonly patients with MG are not able to meet the respiratory demands for sustained physical activities. Respiratory failure, or myasthenic crisis, is the most severe manifestation of respiratory muscle weakness and infections such as bronchopneumonia are common precipitating factors (Thomas et al., 1997). Putman and Wise (1996) reviewed flow volume loops and reported that a relatively high percentage of MG patients with bulbar muscle weakness were at risk for developing upper airway obstruction due to the loss of muscle tone.

Clinical Intervention

There are no specific studies addressing treatment or management of dysphagia for patients with MG. Overall, pharmacologic therapy for the basic disease is the major consideration, with dietary modifications and compensatory maneuvers applied on an individual basis (Palmer et al., 2000). Patients with MG are described as having exercise intolerance and given the pathology present at the NMJ it would appear that inclusion of oral-motor exercises in the treatment plan is contraindicated.

It is imperative that patients who have been identified as having abnormal swallowing be carefully monitored for function and safety. Events that likely would have an innocuous affect on swallowing for individuals without MG, for example stress, fatigue, and minor illness, can completely decompensate a patient with MG. Those identified as being at risk for aspiration and/or nutritional deficiencies related to swallowing should be considered for prophylactic placement of a feeding tube.

Given what is known about the subclinical anomalies in swallowing physiology in patients with MG, a prudent approach to the management of swallowing would include patient and family education early in the course of the disease. Patients should understand what is possible with regard to the impairment, the warning signs for possible dysphagia, and the assessment procedures that are available. Such knowledge may help to prevent complications from developing and perhaps diminish anxiety associated with eating and swallowing. Additionally, reasonable compensations relative to diet adjustments, postures, and eating behavior should be discussed at the first sign of a problem. Finally, given the predilection for patients with MG having esophageal dysfunction, precautions relative to gastroesophageal reflux should be discussed.

Some of the typical, practical guidelines that may be provided to patients with MG include:

- Monitoring strength and fatigue by keeping a log or diary of activities and their affect on the body
- Conserving energy by planning and spacing activities, scheduling rest periods, redesigning work, employing assistive devices, and timing activities to correspond to peak benefits from medications
- Avoiding known triggers that can produce exacerbations of weakness, for example, excessive heat and cold, alcohol, tonic water, or any other substance containing quinine

With regard to swallowing, the following are representative of recommendations provided to patients with MG:

- Eat multiple small meals throughout the day
- Eat larger meals when you have the most energy
- Time meals to correspond to maximum medication benefit
- Sit upright when eating and avoid putting your head back when swallowing
- Avoid large bites of food and attempting to drink liquids rapidly
- Avoid dry food; eat foods moistened with gravy, sauce, broth, butter, sour cream, or yogurt
- Avoid food that crumbles (e.g., crackers, cookies, nuts, chips) or falls apart (e.g., rice)
- Avoid food that requires excessive chewing (e.g., tough meat)
- For some individuals, avoid mixed-consistency foods (e.g., vegetable

soup, dry cereal with milk, fruit salads)

■ Maintain an excellent program of oral hygiene that includes brushing and flossing after meals and cleaning the mouth before eating.

LAMBERT-EATON MYASTHENIC SYNDROME

Lambert-Eaton myasthenic syndrome (LEMS) should be distinguished from MG. In normal function at the level of the NMJ, calcium channels are triggered to open at the presynaptic axon terminal upon arrival of a neural impulse. Calcium ions flow through the voltage regulated channels and facilitate the release of ACh. In LEMS the body's immune system produces calcium channel antibodies that block the opening of calcium channels and thus prevent the release of ACh. Unlike in MG where repetitive contractions result in a progressive reduction in strength, in LEMS repetitive contractions of voluntary muscles will produce a transient increase in muscle strength. In patients with MG the symptoms of muscle weakness tend to develop in a cranial to caudal direction, whereas in LEMS weakness develops from caudal to cranial (Wirtz et al., 2002). LEMS affects autonomic functions as well as skeletal muscles.

LEMS is considered to be quite rare, estimated at 4 cases per one million population. Although it does develop idiopathically, it occurs most commonly in patients with identifiable cancer (e.g., small cell lung carcinoma).

Dysphagia has been reported anecdotally in patients with LEMS (Payne et al., 2005). Because of the impact on the autonomic nervous system, dry mouth is a prominent symptom (O'Neill et al., 1988) and affects swallowing.

The prognosis for patients with LEMS varies depending on the basis for the disease. For those with cancer, particularly small cell lung cancer, the onset of symptoms tends to be rapid and the metastatic disease itself will determine the outcome (Wirtz et al., 2005). Patients without cancer have a more benign course.

SUMMARY

MG is the most common of the neuromuscular diseases occurring at the level of the NMJ. It is a relatively rare chronic autoimmune disease in which the body's own immune system triggers the development of acetylcholine-receptor-specific antibodies that impair Ach receptors on postsynaptic muscle fibers at the level of the NMJ. MG affects voluntary skeletal muscle contractions, especially those that control the eyes, face and oral-pharyngeal functions. When performing repetitive muscle contractions, or when sustained contraction is required to maintain function, for example, lift the eyelids, there is a progressive reduction in muscle strength. For most individuals with MG, pharmacologic therapy involving the use of acetylcholinesterase inhibitors and immunosuppressive drugs is effective. Many patients also undergo surgical removal of the thymus gland, a functional component of the body's immune system that has been implicated in the disease. Although some lifestyle changes are inevitable, most patients with MG can lead relatively normal lives and life expectancy is not reduced.

Up to 25% of patients will experience some degree of dysphagia, which can lead to increased morbidity and mortality. Dysphagia, when present, may affect all stages of swallowing with the most significant and common problems related to chewing, pharyngeal clearance, and airway protection, and esophageal motility. There is evidence for subclinical levels of deglutory muscle weakness that makes individuals with MG susceptible to decompensation from common illnesses, excessive stress, or fatigue. While clinical intervention for dysphagia primarily is dependent on the pharmacologic management of the underlying disease and muscle strengthening exercises are contraindicated, there is a role for the use of dietary modifications and compensatory maneuvers for individuals. Patient and family education regarding safe swallowing and warning signs for dysphagia is important, and prophylactic placement of feeding tubes is warranted in certain cases.

REFERENCES

Beekman, J., Kuks, J. B. M., & Oosterhuis, H. J. G. H. (1997). Myasthenia gravis: Diagnosis and follow-up of 100 consecutive patients. *Journal of Neurology, 244*, 112–118.

Bril, V., & Keshavjee, S. (2007). Management of myasthenia gravis: Does thymectomy provide benefit over medical therapy alone? In M. K. Ferguson (Ed.), *Difficult decisions in thoracic surgery* (pp. 463–468). London, UK: Springer.

Burch, J., Warren-Gash, C., Ingham, V., Patel, M., Bennett, D., & Chaudhuri, K. R. (2006). Myasthenia gravis—a rare presentation with tongue atrophy and fasciculation. *Age and Ageing, 35*, 87–88.

Colton-Hudson, A., Koopman, W. J., Moosa, T., Smith, D., Bach, D., & Nicolle, M. (2002). A prospective assessment of the character-

istics of dysphagia in myasthenia gravis. *Dysphagia, 17*, 147–151.

De Assis, J. L., Marchiori, P. E., & Scaff, M. (1994). Atrophy of the tongue with persistent articulation disorder in myasthenia gravis: Report of 10 patients. *Auris Nasus Larynx, 21*, 215–218.

Ertekin, C., Yuceyar, N., & Aydogdu, I. (1998). Clinical and electrophysiological evaluation of dysphagia in myasthenia gravis. *Journal of Neurology, Neurosurgery and Psychiatry, 65*, 848–856.

Garcia Rio, F., Prados, C., Diez Tejedor, E., Diaz Lobato, S., Alvarez-Sala, R., Villamor, J., & Pino, J. M. (1994). Breathing pattern and central ventilatory drive in mild and moderate generalised myasthenia gravis. *Thorax, 49*, 703–706.

Grob, D., Brunner, N. G., & Namba, T. (1981). The natural course of myasthenia gravis and effect of therapeutic measures. *Annals of the New York Academy of Science, 377*, 652–669.

Heliopoulos, I., Patlakas, G., Vadikolias, K., Artemis, N., K. A. Kleopa, K. A., Maltezos, E., & Piperidou, H. (2003). Maximal voluntary ventilation in myasthenia gravis. *Muscle and Nerve, 27*, 715–719.

Higo, R., Nito, T., & Tayama, N. (2005). Videofluoroscopic assessment of swallowing function in patients with myasthenia gravis. *Journal of the Neurological Sciences, 231*, 45–48.

Huang, M. H., King, K. L., & Chien, K. Y. (1988). Esophageal manometric studies in patients with myasthenia gravis. *Journal of Thoracic and Cardiovascular Surgery, 95*, 281–285.

Jaretzki, A., Barohn, R. J., Ernstoff, R. M., Kaminski, H. J., Keesey, A. S., Penn, A. S., & Sanders, D. B..(2000). Myasthenia gravis: Recommendations for clinical research standards. Task Force of the Medical Scientific Advisory Board of the Myasthenia Gravis Foundation of America. *Neurology, 55*, 16–23.

Keenan, S. P, Alexander, D., Road, J. D., Ryan, C. F., Oger, J., & Wilcox, P. G. (1995). Ventilatory muscle strength and endurance in myasthenia gravis. *European Respiratory Journal, 8,* 1130–1135.

Kluin, K. J., Bromberg, M. B., Feldman, E. L., & Simmons, Z. (1996). Dysphagia in elderly men with myasthenia gravis. *Journal of the Neurological Sciences, 138,* 49–52.

Koopman, W. J., Wiebe, S., Colton-Hudson, A., Moosa, T., Smith, D., Bach, D., & Nicolle, M. W. (2004). Prediction of aspiration in myasthenia gravis. *Muscle and Nerve, 29,* 256–260.

Kramer, P., Atkinson, M., Wyman, S. M., & Ingelfinger, F. J. (1957). The dynamics of swallowing. II: Neuromuscular dysphagia of pharynx. *Journal of Clinical Investigation, 36,* 589–595.

Llabres, M., Molina-Martinez, F. J., & Miralles, F. (2005). Dysphagia as the sole manifestation of myasthenia gravis. *Journal of Neurology, Neurosurgery and Psychiatry, 76,* 1297–1300.

Linke, R., Witt, T. N., & Tatsch, K. (2003). Assessment of esophageal function in patients with myasthenia gravis. *Journal of Neurology, 250,* 601–606.

Nicolle, M. W., Phil, D., Stewart, D. J., Remtulla, H., Chen, R., & Bolton, C. F. (1996). Lambert-Eaton myasthenic syndrome presenting with severe respiratory failure. *Muscle and Nerve, 19,* 1328–1333.

O'Neill, J. H., Murray, N. M. F., & Newsom-Davis, J. (1988). The Lambert-Eaton syndrome: A review of 50 cases. *Brain, 111,* 577–596.

Oosterhuis, H. J. (1989). The natural course of myasthenia gravis: A long-term follow-up study. *Journal of Neurology, Neurosurgery, & Psychiatry, 52,* 1121–1127.

Palmer, J. B., Drennan, J. C., & Baba, M. (2000). Evaluation and treatment of swallowing impairments. *American Family Physician, 61,* 2453–2462.

Payne, S., Wilkins, D., & Howard, R. (2005). An unusual cause of dysphagia. *Journal of Neurology, Neurosurgery, and Psychiatry, 76,* 146.

Putman, M. T., & Wise, R. A. (1996). Myasthenia gravis and upper airway obstruction. *Chest, 109,* 400–404.

Salazar Cabrera, C., de Saa Alvarez Md Mdel, R., Aparicio Pérez, M. S., Marcos Calle, J., & García García, B. (2002). Myasthenia gravis: The otolaryngologist's perspective. *American Journal of Otolaryngology, 23,* 169–172.

Schwab, R. S., & Viets, H. R. (1941). Roentgenoscopy of the pharynx in myasthenia gravis before and after prostigmine injection. *American Journal of Roentgenology, 45,* 357.

Thomas, C. E., Mayer, S. A., Gungor, Y., Swarup, R., Webster E. A., Chang, I., . . . Rowland, L. P. (1997). Myasthenic crisis: clinical features, mortality, complications, and risk factors for prolonged intubation, *Neurology, 48,* 1253–1260.

Weijnen, F. G., Kuks, J. B., van der Bilt, A., van der Glas, H. W., Wassenberg, M. W., & Bosman, F. (2000). Tongue force in patients with myasthenia gravis. *Acta Neurologica Scandinavica, 102,* 303–308.

Wirtz, P. W., Sotodeh, M., Nijnuis, M., van Doorn, P. A., van Engelen, B. G. M., Hintzen, R. Q., . . . Verschuuren, J. J. (2002). Difference in distribution of muscle weakness between myasthenia gravis and the Lambert-Eaton myasthenic syndrome. *Journal of Neurology, Neurosurgery, and Psychiatry, 73,* 766.

Wirtz, P. W., Wintzen, A. R., & Verschuuren, J. J. (2005). Lambert-Eaton myasthenic syndrome has a more progressive course in patients with lung cancer. *Muscle and Nerve, 32,* 226–229.

10 Peripheral Nerve Disease

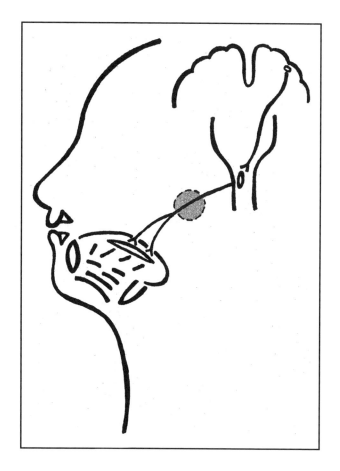

PERIPHERAL NERVES AND NEUROPATHY

A peripheral nerve is classified as either a cranial nerve (CN), emanating from the brainstem, or spinal nerve (SN), arising from the spinal cord. Nerves are found only in the peripheral nervous system (PNS) and are composed of bundles of axons. An axon is a myelin-coated projection from a neuronal cell body that carries impulses to serve either a motor (efferent) or sensory (afferent) function.

A single nerve may include any combination of the following:

- Axons that innervate skeletal muscles to provide for voluntary movement
- Axons that innervate visceral organs and glands for involuntary, autonomic control
- Axons that carry sensory information that originated in either the external environment (e.g., sensory receptors in skin, eyes and ears) or internal environment (muscle, joints, and visceral organs) to the central nervous system (CNS).

Peripheral neuropathy represents a pathologic process that affects peripheral nerves and can cause impairments that are manifested in any of the functions served by the damaged axons. Impairment may involve multiple nerves, referred to as *polyneuropathy*, or a single nerve, designated as *mononeuropathy*. With regard to skeletal muscles, neuropathies can result in paresis or paralysis. Functionally, an individual may lose the ability to walk or grasp objects when the efferent axons of spinal nerves are involved; limit speech, swallowing, and/or the ability to move the eyes when efferent axons in cranial nerves are affected; or experience symptoms such as blurred vision, urinary incontinence and fainting if efferent autonomic fibers are involved. Among the symptoms of sensory axon neuropathy are pain, tingling, numbness, or burning sensations.

The axons of peripheral nerves are components of lower motor neurons (LMNs), with a cell body of the projecting neuron at the proximal end and a neuromuscular junction (NMJ) at the distal end (Figure 10–1). The symptoms experienced by any individual patient depend

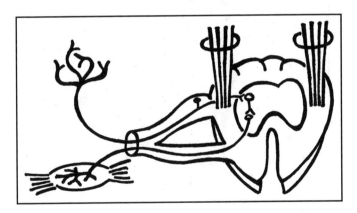

Figure 10–1. The lower motor neuron. As depicted here, a lower motor neuron is composed of a cell body located in the gray matter of the spinal cord, an axon extending out along the anterior root and into a spinal nerve, and neuromuscular junctions on muscle fibers. Impulses may be generated by action potentials arriving from sensory neurons, as in sensory-motor reflexes, or from descending upper motor neurons, as in voluntary actions. The same basic design also exists at the level of the brainstem.

entirely on the specific nerves affected, the pattern of nerve involvement and the underlying cause of the neuropathy. Pathology that affects a peripheral nerve can occur at various sites:

- At the cell body—generally involving either motor neurons and causing motor neuron disease, described in Chapter 11, or sensory neurons producing either sensory neuronopathy or dorsal root ganglionopathy
- Along axonal fibers (axonopathy)—a condition in which the cell bodies remain intact, but axons are affected in proportion to their length (longer axons being most prone to degeneration)
- In the myelin sheath (demyelinating neuropathies)—damaging the myelin protein sheath of axons and impairing the propagation of impulses along the axon.

CLASSIFICATION OF PERIPHERAL NEUROPATHIES

There are a number of conditions that can cause peripheral neuropathy some of which are acquired, for example trauma and toxin exposure, whereas others are inherited, such as Charcot-Marie-Tooth disease. The following outline lists most types of peripheral neuropathy classified by cause with examples for each:

- Physical trauma—compression from casts or splints, accidents, slipped discs between vertebrae; and surgical injury as found following carotid endarterectomy or anterior approach cervical spine fusion

- Systemic or metabolic disorders—kidney disorders leading to the buildup of toxins; hormonal imbalances like hypothyroidism causing tissue swelling that exerts constant pressure on peripheral nerves or acromegaly resulting in abnormal enlargement of boney structures that can compress nerves; vitamin deficiencies (particularly E, B1, B6, B12, and niacin); excessive alcohol consumption causing alcohol neuropathy; chronically high blood sugar levels, and/or neurovascular changes as seen in diabetes are particularly harmful to peripheral nerves; and cancer which can produce a tumor that infiltrates a nerve, exerts pressure on nerve fibers or triggers a paraneoplastic syndrome causing widespread peripheral nerve damage.
- Toxins and drugs—heavy metals such as lead, arsenic and mercury may be inhaled or ingested to cause nerve damage; drugs like vincristine and certain chemotherapeutic agents have also been implicated in neuropathy.
- Inflammatory disorders—acute inflammatory demyelinating neuropathy, also known as Guillain-Barré syndrome, and chronic inflammatory demyelinating polyneuropathy (CIDP) are examples of conditions where protective tissues surrounding peripheral nerves are damaged and can lead to pathology of the nerve fibers themselves; autoimmune inflammatory disorders like Sjögren syndrome and systemic lupus erythematosus can cause impairment at several levels including the CNS, peripheral nerves, NMJ, and the muscle; and sarcoidosis,

a multisystem granulomatous inflammatory disease can be the basis for a neuropathy, myopathy, or obstruction that leads to dysphagia.

■ Infections—HIV infection, hepatitis, diphtheria, Lyme disease, and shingles have the potential to cause peripheral neuropathy.

■ Genetic diseases—the pathogenesis of Friedreich ataxia commonly results from impairment of central neural fibers like the spinocerebellar tracts, as well as peripheral nerve damage; and Charcot-Marie-Tooth disease, also known as hereditary motor and sensory neuropathy (HMSN), is an inherited condition most often associated with loss of muscle tissue and sensation in the feet and legs, but in certain forms will cause degeneration of cranial nerves.

■ Generally, the longer the nerve the more susceptible it is to damage from the processes that cause peripheral neuropathy. For that reason, CN involvement is less common than SN pathology and pharyngeal muscles thus are seldom impaired (Dyck, Prineas, & Pollard, 1993; Ropper, 1986).

Worldwide, the most common etiology for peripheral neuropathy is diabetes. Although it is beyond the scope of this chapter to thoroughly review all of the mechanisms contributing to the pathogenesis of diabetic neuropathy, it is important to recognize that there many causative mechanisms at play. Although the neuropathic processes are not completely understood, they tend to fall into two categories: disturbances in neuronal cell metabolism and ischemia. With regard to cell metabolism, the underlying prob-

lem may in part be attributed to hyperglycemic-induced oxidative stress causing damage to DNA and cell membranes, ultimately culminating in neuron degeneration. The second pathological mechanism, nerve ischemia, occurs as a consequence of damage to the walls of the small blood vessels that nourish axons. The degree of skin deinnervation is directly related to the duration and severity of diabetes. A further complication for patients with diabetes is that they appear to be more prone to developing pressure induced neuropathies, for example, carpal tunnel syndrome, than nondiabetic individuals. Furthermore, other causes of polyneuropathy also may be present in a given individual, for example, alcoholism, vitamin deficiency, and drug-induced neuropathy. All of these factors, together with several other pathologic processes, many of which are not completely defined, contribute to diabetic polyneuropathy.

Interestingly, patients with diabetic polyneuropathy often experience symmetric symptoms, generally beginning in the feet before progressing to more proximal parts of the lower extremities. This is referred to as a "length-dependent pattern" of degeneration and is also found in other forms of peripheral neuropathy.

Some neuropathies impair nerve fibers independent of length and may therefore affect bulbar musculature more frequently. Specifically, patients with Guillain-Barré syndrome commonly have CN involvement with dysphagia as a symptom. Less commonly, a class of disorders referred to as *chronic acquired demyelinating polyneuropathies* (CADP) can present with bulbar muscle impairment, most likely CN VII with facial muscle paralysis, but rarely with CN IX, X, and XII affected (Dyck et al., 1993). Charcot-Marie-Tooth disease is the most common inherited peripheral neuropathy, and although variants of this disease can cause dysphagia, it is rare that cranial nerves are involved (Roa et al., 1993).

Anecdotal reports of dysphagia have been documented for many conditions for which PN pathology is the level of dysfunction. Although no one disease can be representative for all cases where peripheral neuropathy is the basis for impairment, the following description of Guillain-Barré syndrome should help guide clinicians when treating patients with peripheral nerve involvement.

GUILLAIN-BARRÉ SYNDROME

Definition

Guillain-Barré syndrome (GBS) is one of the autoimmune conditions in which multiple motor, sensory and autonomic peripheral nerves, are attacked. Generally, the first symptoms are weakness and sensory changes, for example, tingling or numbness, in the lower extremities. This frequently progresses from the legs to the upper extremities and can eventually involve nerves that support respiration and bulbar functions like speech and swallowing. The progression of symptoms can develop within hours, but more commonly over the course of days to a few weeks. Commonly, the onset of symptoms develops within a few days or weeks following a viral infection of the respiratory or gastrointestinal system, and more rarely can be triggered by surgical procedures or vaccinations.

GBS is considered to be a syndrome and not a disease because it involves a collection of symptoms and no known

disease-causing agent has been identified. It is also referred to as *acute inflammatory demyelinating polyneuropathy* (AIDP), *acute polyradiculoneuropathy*, or *polyradiculoneuritis*. In 1916, the French physicians Georges Guillain, Jean-Alexandre Barré, and André Strohl described a series of patients with symptoms similar to acute paralytic syndrome, or *poliomyelitis*, a common and dreaded neurologic condition of the time. In this new syndrome, later to be labeled GBS, there was a differential finding of increased protein in the cerebrospinal fluid (CSF) with an absence of increased white blood cells. Although GBS is variable in its presentation, progressing at different rates, with different patterns of progression and degrees of recovery, it appears without warning and usually abates spontaneously. Another related, but distinct syndrome known as *chronic inflammatory demyelinating polyneuropathy* (CIDP) is marked by a slowly progressive motor and sensory neuropathy of the arms and legs followed by either spontaneous recovery or a relapse-remitting course.

The commonality for these particular immunologic inflammatory conditions is the breakdown of myelin and, in severe cases, the degeneration of axons. Damage to myelin can lead to segmental demyelination, or the loss of myelin over a few segments of the axon. Myelin is a lipid and protein-based electrical insulation that is formed by *Schwann cells* in the PNS (*oligodendrocytes* provide myelin in the CNS). As shown in Figure 10–2, myelin coating is segmented along the length of an axon with gaps called nodes of Ranvier. Nerve impulses propagated along a large-diameter myelinated axon can be propagated about 5,000 times faster than along unmyelinated fibers, and the insulation prevents impulses from escaping

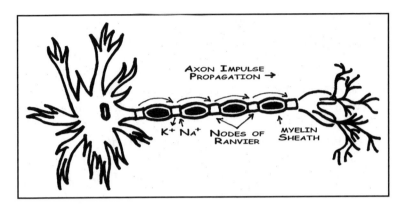

Figure 10–2. Neuron with myelinated axon. Segmented myelin coating along the length of an axon allows neural impulses to jump from one node of Ranvier to the next at much greater speeds than unmyelinated axons.

the axon (Hartline & Colman, 2007). Impulses literally jump from node to node in myelinated axons, whereas they move along more slowly in a wavelike fashion in unmyelinated fibers. Many diseases and conditions are considered to be demyelinating. Multiple sclerosis, transverse myelitis, leukoencephalopathy, and leukodystrophy are all demyelinating diseases of the CNS. Conditions such as diphtheria, Charcot-Marie-Tooth disease, CIDP, GBS, and heavy metal poisoning, for example, lead, arsenic, and mercury, commonly result in peripheral neuropathy.

Signs and Diagnostic Criteria

There is great variability in the presentation of symptoms in GBS. Hughes and Cornblath (2005) describe at least four subtypes of acute peripheral neuropathy that can occur. Typically, initial symptoms are:

■ Sensory—pain, numbness, pins-and-needles paresthesia in the extremities

■ Motor—weakness either proximal, distal or some combination in the limbs; facial muscle weakness and other bulbar and ocular motor nerve involvement; respiratory muscle weakness sufficient to require ventilatory support (Hughes & Cornblath, 2005)

■ Autonomic—commonly urine retention, ileus, sinus tachycardia, hypertension, cardiac arrhythmia, and postural hypotension (Hughes and Cornblath, 2005).

The diagnostic criteria established by Asbury and Cornblath (1990) include:

■ Loss of deep tendon reflexes in involved limbs
■ Slowing nerve conduction velocity (NCV) on electrophysiologic testing
■ Excessive protein found in cerebrospinal fluid.

The diagnosis also is made largely on the basis of clinical presentation with the inexplicable neuropathy reaching a peak in less than four weeks, and the presence of weakness and diminished or absent reflexes. Differential diagnosis of acute flaccid paralysis requires recognition that the problem is indeed at the level of the PN and not in the brainstem or spinal cord. Among the "rule-outs" are: stroke or encephalitis in the brainstem, acute poliomyelitis, acute myelopathy from a space occupying lesion or transverse myelitis, myasthenia gravis, muscle disorders, and biological or industrial toxins. Additionally, other etiologies for peripheral neuropathy must be ruled out, particularly, post-rabies vaccine neuropathy, heavy metal poisoning, diphtheritic neuropathy, and vasculitic neuropathy (Asbury & Cornblath, 1990).

Evolution

For most patients with GBS, the disease reaches its peak at 2 weeks and almost certainly by 4 weeks. The plateau phase is unpredictable, lasting anywhere from a few days to several months before recovery begins. Ventilation is required in about 33% of cases. The recovery sequence generally follows a predictable pattern that begins with proximal gains in strength followed by distal return. In severe cases, muscle atrophy will be evident within 2 weeks of paralysis, but upon recovery muscle bulk generally returns. Mortality is between 4 and 15% of patients during the acute bout of neuropathy, and up to 20% remain disabled after a year (Rees, Thompson, Smeeton, & Hughes, 1998). Even after what appears to be full recovery, residual weakness and fatigue frequently persist, explained by the documented loss of motor units on electrophysiologic exam-

ination (Merkies, Schmitz, Samijn, van der Meché, & van Doorn, 1999).

Although most patients make a good recovery from GBS, a poorer prognosis has been linked to the following variables (Hughes & Cornblath, 2005; Hughes, Greenwood, Perkin, & Healy, 1985; Visser, Schmitz, Meulstee, van Doorn, & van der Meché, 1999; Winer):

- Elderly patients (children tend to recover rapidly and completely)
- Rapid onset
- Need for ventilation support
- Failure to improve within three weeks of reaching peak deficit
- Prolonged immobility
- Low amplitude or absent motor responses
- Preceding illness marked by diarrhea
- Presence of cytomegalovirus.

Epidemiology

Most reports suggest that GBS occurs at a median rate of about 1.3 cases per 100,000 people per year (Hughes & Rees, 1997). Men are one and one-half times more likely to be diagnosed with the syndrome than women, and older individuals are more likely to be affected (Hughes & Cornblath, 2005). Although most cases are sporadic, there have been clusters associated with bacterial enteritis caused by water contamination (Hughes, Hadden, Gregson, & Smith, 1999). About two-thirds of all patients report having had flulike symptoms or gastroenteritis within the previous 6 weeks. After swine flu vaccinations in the United States in 1976, fear arose because of a slight increase in incidence of GBS. However, other influenza vaccines have not been associated with the same level of risk. Analysis of risk between 1992 and 1994 suggested an increase of about one case per million vaccinations (Lasky et al., 1998).

Medical/Surgical Treatment

Because the onset and evolution of symptoms in GBS is highly variable and the need for intubation and ventilatory support can be precipitous, most patients with GBS need to be admitted to a tertiary care center with an appropriately staffed intensive-care unit available. Close observation and anticipation of complications such as circulatory instability and autonomic dysfunction are necessary to improve the chances for a favorable outcome. Two primary modalities of treatment have been used to minimize the impact of GBS and speed recovery: plasmapheresis and high-dose intravenous immunoglobulin (IVIg).

Plasmapheresis, also referred to as plasma exchange, involves the separation of the fluid component of the blood, or plasma, from blood cells (red cells, white cells, and platelets). This process is performed by use of a cell separator, usually either a device that spins blood at high speed to separate cells from fluid or filtering through a membrane that only allows the fluid component of blood to pass through. In large studies plasmapheresis, when performed within the first 2 weeks, resulted in more rapid recovery as measured by reducing the number of days on ventilation by about one-half (24 vs. 48 days) and the number of days to ambulation (53 vs. 85 days). When plasma exchange was begun after 2 weeks, treatment was ineffective. When evaluated at one-year postonset, more patients who had been treated by plasma exchange

recovered full strength, 71% of treated patients versus 52% of controls (Hahn, 1998). Plasmapheresis is not completely without risk, especially for patients with unstable circulatory systems. About 10% of patients can develop worsening of symptoms within 1 or 2 weeks of treatment and between 4 and 10% of patients have contraindications for this treatment, for example, severe homeostasis abnormalities, unstable hemodynamics, or uncontrolled sepsis (Raphaël, Chevret, Harboun, & Jars-Guincestre, 2001).

High-dose intravenous immunoglobulin (IVIg) therapy provides the patient with a blood product that has been extracted from the plasma of numerous donors. This is a form of replacement therapy in which purified human plasma is used to trigger an immune response in the hope that it will inhibit production of pathologic antibodies that precipitated the syndrome. In a randomized controlled trial, IVIg therapy was compared to plasma exchange and combined treatment in three groups of patients. Using a 7-point disability scale, blinded observers found no differences between the groups (Hughes, Raphaël, Swan, & van Doorn, 2006). Most studies have found that patient recovery using IVIg was equal to that of plasma exchange, but with the added advantage of being safer to administer.

Swallowing in Guillain-Barré Syndrome

Epidemiology

Bulbar symptoms are not rare in patients with GBS and there are variants of the syndrome in which it is more common, for example, a pharyngeal-cervical-brachial variant (Murakami et al., 2006). In fact, there is evidence to suggest that the presence of certain antibodies contribute to the specific neuropathy in a given patient. For example, higher levels of the anti-GT1a antibody may contribute to a slightly higher incidence in dysphagia (Ilyas et al, 1998). Although bulbar symptoms, including dysphagia, are rarely the initial neurologic sign (Ropper, 1986), bulbar weakness has been found in up to 57% of patients in one study (Ng et al., 1995). One variant of GBS, Miller-Fisher syndrome (MFS), characterized by ataxia, ophthalmoplegia, and areflexia, is often accompanied by involvement of medullary cranial nerves, especially involving facial palsy (Mori, Kuwabara, Fukutake, Yuki, & Hattori, 2001). In a series of 8 cases with MFS variant, 6 had facial palsy, 6 had dysphagia, and 3 required ventilation support (Rodríguez Uranga et al., 2004).

Given that GBS presents with great variability in terms of severity and neurologic involvement, it follows that swallowing impairments will likewise be extremely variable. Furthermore, the presence of severe dysphagia during the course of GBS, especially in the later stages, will be more likely to have some degree of residual impairment following recovery. Fortunately, swallowing function does recover fully in the majority of cases.

Physiology

In the evolution of symptoms about one-third of patients will experience a rapid decline in vital capacity to the point that they will require mechanical ventilation. This often is accompanied by ineffective cough and bulbar muscle weakness, the combination of which functionally impairs the ability to swallow. The characteristics of a swallowing impairment will depend entirely on the status of the respiratory system and on which combination of cranial nerves and associated bulbar muscles are involved, and to what extent. For example, the motor branch of the trigeminal nerve controls both muscles of mastication and mylohyoid function, with lesions thus impairing both chewing and laryngeal elevation during swallows. The facial nerves are critical for important aspects of oral stage swallowing, including the motor input required to achieve lip seal and major aspects of taste sensation and saliva production. Branches of the glossopharyngeal and vagus nerves serve many important sensory and motor functions that are critical to swallowing and dysphagia symptoms will reflect the specific nerve pathology. The hypoglossal nerve controls tongue movement that is critical to the oral and early-to-middle pharyngeal stages of swallowing.

Chen and colleagues (1996) reported on 14 patients with GBS seen for videofluoroscopic swallowing evaluation over a 5-year period. Ten of their patients had combined oral and pharyngeal stage abnormalities, with the remaining four demonstrating only pharyngeal dysfunction. The severity range for these 14 patients also varied from mild to severe. Fortunately, most patients, even those with severe impairments, recovered within four to five weeks. One patient, however, continued to display severe deficits for 6 weeks and even at 8 weeks postonset had a moderate degree of impairment. Some residual swallowing impairments may be detected by careful examination even after patients are well into the recovery phase of the syndrome. The authors note that, although no patient in their series developed aspiration pneumonia, the risk for this complication remains high. It appears clear from reports such as this, and from clinical experience, that swallowing abnormalities in GBS are not homogeneous and clinical presentations vary in terms of severity and motor-sensory characteristics.

Clinical Intervention

In all but the mildest cases, patients with GBS are first encountered in the intensive care unit. Initial clinical examination begins with a careful history and a description of the patient's subjective impression of swallowing and oral-motor functions. A detailed structural-functional examination of the swallowing musculature will provide valuable baseline data that can be used to track either the patient's course of progression or recovery. Assessment of the respiratory system as it supports both speech and swallowing is critical for any patient with progressive weakness that involves cervical spinal nerves and/or cranial nerves. For the speech-language pathologist this assessment procedure is outlined in Chapter 5. Indications for instrumental assessment, particularly videofluoroscopic evaluation, are likely to exist for those patients who have experienced swallowing difficulties during the course of the syndrome. These assessments generally are performed during either the plateau or recovery phase of GBS. For those who are recovering from bulbar impairments and swallowing function is beginning to return, endoscopic swallowing examinations can be valuable in helping to determine the patient's readiness to begin oral feeding. Additionally, clinical signs such as the volume and quality of the patient's phonation, the precision of motor speech movements, and the patient's ability to manage oral secretions are important indicators for both progression of symptoms and recovery of function.

During the progressive phase, it is not uncommon for patients to undergo tracheostomy to facilitate ventilation support. Nasal-gastric feeding or gastrostomy tube feeding may be required to provide alternative routes for nutrition and hydration. Intervention during this phase is focused on frequent clinical re-assessment to monitor the status of swallowing and adjust management interventions accordingly. Because the progressive phase often is marked by a preciptious decline in function, and swallowing difficulties often are overshadowed by the deterioration of respiratory functions, videofluoroscopic examinations during this phase are infrequently performed.

When a patient reaches the plateau phase, the clinician's tactics often change to providing more of an intensive treatment approach. Dikeman and Kazandjian (2010) recently published guidelines for managing dysphagia in GBS that included the following areas of focus: (1) oromotor strengthening through isometric and resistance exercises, (2) cough retraining, (3) implementation of compensatory maneuvers and postural modifications, and (4) diet modification once oral intake has been reestablished. Although these interventions have not been specifically investigated for patients with GBS, exercises targeting particular muscles and utilizing methods that conform to the principles of exercise physiology appear have a strong physiologic basis. For example, investigators have reported promising results after using a spring-loaded one-way valve to overload expiratory muscles and improve the "cough volume acceleration" and other parameters that relate to the efficiency and effectiveness of airway clearance (Pitts et al., 2009). There is good rationale for applying this during the recovery phase of GBS. With regard to the use of maneuvers and postures, specific application would depend on the individual patient and what they were able to demonstrate during instrumental examinations as being appropriate compensations. However, there is a potential role for maneuvers such as the Mendelsohn and supraglottic swallow, and for neck-flexed or head-turn postures.

Importantly, instrumental assessments are utilized to determine the specific compensatory maneuvers, postures, and diet textures that can be employed to facilitate swallowing safety and efficiency. Dikeman and Kazandjian (2010) emphasize that dysphagia treatment should be integrated into a comprehensive rehabilitation program that includes physical, occupational, and respiratory therapy with attention to chest physiotherapy, mobilization, and proper positioning. It is important to be aware that the effects of position on the respiratory system can vary, depending on the specific underlying neuromuscular impairments (see Chapter 5).

Because cognitive functions are not considered to be a component of GBS, these patients generally are able to learn and effectively employ compensatory controls that allow them to better protect their airway and swallow more efficiently. Biofeedback techniques such as sEMG, pharyngeal manometry, and nasopharyngeal endoscopy, although not specifically studied for this population, potentially could improve swallowing by allowing for higher level cortical control over the process. Given the enormous variation in type, severity, and distribution of peripheral nerve impairment in GBS, the treatment approach for each patient must be based on individual characteristics and applied at an appropriate point during the course of the disease.

SUMMARY

Peripheral neuropathies are motor and/or sensory impairments caused by conditions affecting the axons of spinal and/or cranial nerves. There are myriad conditions that can cause peripheral neuropathy and they fall into categories of trauma, metabolic disorders, drugs and toxins, inflammatory diseases, infections, and genetic disorders. The most common specific etiology of peripheral neuropathy is diabetes, a condition that impairs the metabolism of the neuron and results in ischemia. GBS is an example of an inflammatory disorder causing acute pathology of peripheral nerves. It is an autoimmune based syndrome, often preceded by a viral infection and characterized by a relatively precipitous onset of symptoms. Motor weakness and sensory tingling and numbness may develop over a few hours, days, or even weeks. Although there is great variability in the presentation and progression, GBS commonly begins in the lower extremities, advances to involve the arms, and in about a third of cases will impair respiratory function to the degree that the patient will require mechanical ventilation. In the typical case, the acute neurologic impairment reaches a peak at 2 weeks, the symptoms plateau for a few days to weeks, and then recovery begins in a predictable pattern of proximal improvement followed by distal muscle function. Although largely dependent on the availability and quality of intensive care, about 90% of patients survive the acute phase the majority makes a near full recovery within a year. There are, however, a significant number of patients who will have residual weakness and fatigue beyond a year. Certain variants of this syndrome are more commonly associated with bulbar symptoms and are thus more likely to experience dysphagia. When swallowing problems develop, the characteristics will be entirely dependent on the specific cranial nerves that have been affected and on the concomitant impairment in respiratory function. Oral and pharyngeal stage swallowing abnormalities have been described in a high percentage of patients with GBS, but the characteristics are not homogeneous. Interventions are by necessity individualized according to the specific impairments, but may involve oral-motor strengthening, cough retraining, and dietary modifications. Because these patients generally retain higher level cognitive functions, the utilization of biofeedback for retraining and implementation of compensatory postures and maneuvers may be beneficial.

REFERENCES

Asbury, A. K., & Cornblath, D. R. (1990). Assessment of current diagnostic criteria for Guillain-Barré syndrome. *Annals of Neurology, 27*, S21–S24.

Chen, M. Y. M., Donofrio, P. D., Frederick, M. G., Ott, D. J., & Pikna, L. A. (1996). Videofluoroscopic evaluation of patients with Guillain-Barré syndrome. *Dysphagia, 11,* 11–13.

Dikeman, K. J., & Kazandjian, M. S. (2010). Guillain Barré syndrome. In H. N. Jones & J. C. Rosenbek (Eds.), *Dysphagia in rare conditions: An Encyclopedia* (pp. 243–248). San Diego, CA: Plural.

Dyck, P. J., Prineas, J., & Pollard, J. (1993). Chronic inflammatory demyelinating polyradiculoneuropathy. In: P. J. Dyck, P. K., Thomas, J. W. Griffin, P. A. Low, & J. F. Poduslo (Eds.), *Peripheral neuropathy* (3rd ed., pp. 1498–1517). Philadelphia, PA: W. B. Saunders.

Hahn, A. F. (1998). Guillain-Barré syndrome. *Lancet, 352,* 635–641.

Hartline, D. K., & Colman, D. R. (2007). Rapid conduction and the evolution of giant axons and myelinated fibers. *Current Biology, 17,* R29–R35.

Hughes, R. A. C., & Cornblath, D. R. (2005). Guillain-Barré syndrome. *Lancet, 366,* 1653–1666.

Hughes, R. A. C., Hadden, R. D. M., Gregson, N. A., & Smith, K. J. (1999). Pathogenesis of Guillain-Barré syndrome. *Journal of Neuroimmunology, 100,* 74–97.

Hughes, R. A. C., Raphaël, J. C., Swan, A. V., & van Doorn, P. A. (2006). Intravenous immunoglobulin for Guillain-Barré syndrome. *Cochrane Database of Systematic Reviews 2006, Issue 1.* Art. No.: CD002063.

Hughes, R. A. C., & Rees, J. H. (1997). Clinical and epidemiologic features of Guillain-Barré syndrome. *Journal of Infectious Diseases, 176,* S92–S98.

Ilyas, A. A., Cook, S. D., Mithen, F. A., Taki, T., Kasama, T., Handa, S., . . . Lif, Y.-T. (1998). Antibodies to GT1a ganglioside in patients with Guillain-Barré syndrome. *Journal of Neuroimmunology, 82,* 160–167.

Lasky, T., Terracciano, G. J., Magder, L., Koski, C. L., Ballesteros, M., Nash, D., . . . Chen, R. T. (1998). The Guillain-Barré syndrome and the 1992–1993 and 1993–1994 influenza vaccines. *New England Journal of Medicine, 339,* 1797–1802.

Merkies, I. S. P., Schmitz, I. Samijn, J. P., van der Meché, F. G. & van Doorn, P. A. (1999). Fatigue in immune-mediated polyneuropathies. *Neurology, 53,* 1648–1654.

Mori, M., Kuwabara, S., Fukutake, T., Yuki, N., & Hattori, T. (2001). Clinical features and prognosis of Miller-Fisher syndrome. *Neurology, 56,* 1104–1106.

Murakami, N., Tomita, Y., Koga, M., Takahashi, E., Katada, Y., Sakuta, R., & Nagal, T. (2006). An adolescent with pharyngeal-cervical-brachial variant of Guillain-Barré syndrome after cytomegalovirus infection. *Brain and Development, 28,* 269–271.

Ng, K. K. P., Howard, R. S., Fish, D. R., Hirsch, N. P., Wiles, C. M., Murray, N. M. F., & Miller,

D. H. (1995). The management and outcome of severe Guillain-Barré syndrome. *Quarterly Journal of Medicine, 88*, 243–250.

Pitts, T., Bolser, D., Rosenbek, J., Troche, M., Okun, M., & Sapienza, C. M. (2009). Impact of expiratory muscle strength training on voluntary cough and swallow function in Parkinson's disease. *Chest, 135*, 1301–1308.

Raphaël, J. C., Chevret, S., Harboun, M., & Jars-Guincestre, M-C. (2001). Intravenous immune globulins in patients with Guillain-Barré syndrome and contraindications to plasma exchange: 3 days versus 6 days. *Journal of Neurology, Neurosurgery and Psychiatry, 71*, 235–238.

Rees, J. H., Thompson, R. D., Smeeton, N. C., & Hughes, R. A. C. (1998). An epidemiological study of Guillain-Barré syndrome in South East England. *Journal of Neurology, Neurosurgery and Psychiatry, 64*, 74–77.

Roa, B. B., Garcia, C. A., Suter, U., Kulpa, D. A., Wise, C. A., Mueller, J., . . . Lupski, J. R. (1993). Charcot-Marie-Tooth disease type 1A: Association with a spontaneous point mutation in the PMP22 gene. *New England Journal of Medicine, 329*, 96–101.

Rodríguez Uranga, J. J., Delgado López, F., Franco Macías, E., Sánchez Arjona, M. B., Martínez Quesada, C., & Palomino García, A. (2004). Miller-Fisher syndrome: Clinical features, associated infections and clinical course in 8 cases. *Medical Clinics (Barcelona), 122*, 223–226.

Ropper, A. H. (1986). Unusual clinical variants and signs in Guillain-Barré syndrome. *Archives of Neurology, 43*, 1150–1152.

Visser, L. H., Schmitz, P. I. M., Meulstee, J. P., van Doorn, A., & van der Meché, F. G. A. (1999). Prognostic factors of Guillain-Barré syndrome after intravenous immunoglobulin or plasma exchange. *Neurology, 53*, 598–604.

Winer, J. B., Hughes, R. A., Greenwood, R. J., Perkin, G. C., & Healy, M. J., (1985). Prognosis in Guillain-Barré syndrome. *Lancet, 25*, 1202–1203.

11 Motor Neuron Disease

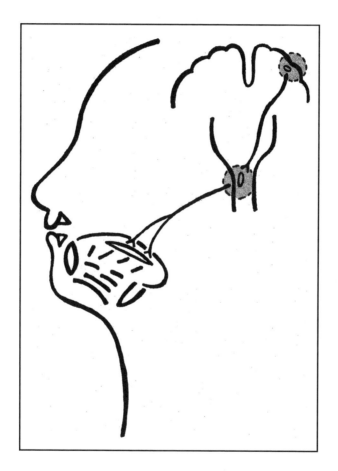

MOTOR NEURONS

A motor neuron is an efferent cell found in the nervous system that either directly or indirectly activates the contraction of muscles or controls their tone and move-

ment. The motor neurons that are of concern in this chapter communicate with muscles that are under voluntary control of the central nervous system (CNS) and do not necessarily activate visceral muscle contractions. There principally are two types of motor neurons, upper and lower. Upper motor neurons (UMNs) send impulses from higher levels of the nervous system, primarily from the forebrain, to neuronal cells located in lower levels of the CNS, specifically the brainstem and spinal cord. Lower motor neurons (LMNs) residing in the gray matter of the brainstem and spinal cord are activated and modulated by upper motor neurons. LMNs, via their axons, carry impulses to voluntary muscles and act as the "final common pathway" for muscle innervation.

UMNs are classified as either *pyramidal* or *extrapyramidal* and, respectively, send their signals to LMNs either directly or indirectly. Soma of pyramidal neurons in the cereboral cortex contribute axons to corticobulbular and corticospinal tracts, pathways of myelinated axons that descend directly to the brainstem and spinal cord to communicate with lower motor neurons. This *direct activation pathway* generally is associated with conscious, skilled movements. All other UMN tracts are considered to be *indirect activation pathways*. They originate from other regions of the forebrain and brainstem and descend to influence LMNs and their corresponding muscles for more autonomous actions. That is, these motor neurons are concerned with unconscious adjustments in skeletal muscles to influence reflex actions, balance, and posture. Examples of these extrapyramidal pathways are the tectospinal, rubrospinal, vestibulospinal, and reticulospinal tracts.

In optimal function, LMNs receive a constant flow of signals from UMN pathways, both direct and indirect. In turn, the LMNs transmit a steady stream of impulses to skeletal muscle fibers for automatic adjustments in tone and posture and to initiate purposeful muscle contractions. Thus, both the direct and indirect UMN pathways must be operating optimally to provide LMNs with a balanced flow of impulses. And in turn, LMNs must transmit proper information to muscles to ensure a state of readiness from which skilled, voluntary movements can be initiated.

MOTOR NEURON DISEASES

Motor neuron disease (MND) refers to the group of progressive disorders that are characterized by destruction of motor neurons, that is, UMNs and/or LMNs. There are four types of adult onset MND as seen in Table 11–1. The most common type of MND is amyotrophic lateral sclerosis (ALS).

ALS, also known as Lou Gehrig disease in the United States, is a progressive disease characterized by degeneration of UMNs, corticobulbar and/or corticospinal tracts, and LMNs, neurons originating in the brainstem and spinal cord. ALS is characterized by an initial focal degeneration of nerve cells that control voluntary and involuntary muscle movement with subsequent rapid degeneration that spreads to other regions of the body. The degeneration occurs in the pyramidal neurons (Betz cells, 5th layer of cerebral cortex) of the precentral gyrus (area 4, motor cortex) and alpha motor neurons from the brainstem and spinal cord (Rocha, Reis, Simoes, Fonseca, & Mendes Ribeiro, 2005). The precise etiology or pathophysiologic mechanism is unknown. Symptoms of classic ALS often begin in the limbs, for example, weakness in one or more extremities. However, it also may begin in the bulbar region, that is, muscles for speech and swallowing; in this case, it frequently is called progres-

Table 11–1. Four Types of Adult Onset Motor Neuron Disease (MND)

Type	Classic Amyotrophic Lateral Sclerosis (ALS)	Progressive Muscle Atrophy (PMA)	Progressive Bulbar Palsy (PBP)	Primary Lateral Sclerosis (PLS)
Motor neuron neurologic signs	UMN & LMN	LMN only	UMN &/or LMN	UMN only may or may not progress to diagnosis of ALS. If only UMN signs for ≥4 years, likely to be pure PLS (Gordon et al., 2006)
Muscle involvement	Bulbar & Spinal	Spinal (Rarely, bulbar)	Bulbar only	Bulbar & Spinal
Prognosis	Median survival 4.32 years (Czaplinski, Yen, Simpson, & Appel, 2006)	Longer than ALS	Median survival 2–3 years (Leigh et al., 2003)	Survival much longer than ALS. Higher levels of independence for years or decades (Gordon et al., 2006)

sive bulbar palsy (PBP). Onset of ALS in muscles for respiration occurs rarely, as it accounts for less than 3% of ALS cases (Gautier et al., 2009).

Primary lateral sclerosis (PLS) is a relatively rare form of MND, characterized by UMN involvement only. Clinically, "pure" PLS is defined as UMN involvement on diagnosis, with no evidence of LMN involvement for a period of at least 4 years (Gordon et al., 2006). Initially and otherwise, this condition can be referred to as UMN dominant ALS. PLS most often occurs with limb onset symptoms, but can occur with bulbar onset as well (Gordon, Cheng, Katz, Mitsumoto, & Rowland, 2009). Owing to the UMN involve-

ments, spasticity is common and LMN signs such as atrophy and fasciculations do not occur in this group. Survival is much longer in this group, and individuals with this diagnosis can maintain higher levels of independence for years. Although the prognosis differs from classic ALS, the same principles of assessment and management described below for ALS apply.

Progressive bulbar palsy (PBP) is a type of MND, and more specifically, a form of bulbar-onset ALS or PLS (Caroscio, Mulvihill, Sterling, & Abrams, 1987; Pascuzzi, 2002). For those who survive the initial bulbar degeneration, it nearly always progresses to classic ALS, as it spreads to the limbs and thorax (Karam, Scelsa, & Macgowan, 2010). Rarely, it can progress to PLS (Gordon et al., 2009). Some divide PBP into two categories (Francis, Bach, & DeLisa, 1999): progressive bulbar palsy (LMN form) and progressive pseudobulbar palsy (UMN form). Most often, PBP develops like ALS with a combination of UMN and LMN involvement (Francis et al., 1999; Rocha et al., 2005; Strong & Rosenfeld, 2003).

In PBP, the focal degeneration in the pyramidal system involves the lowest portion of the precentral gyrus and the descending corticobulbar tract. Once the disease spreads to include the higher portions of the precentral gyrus and corticospinal tract, it likely would be considered classic ALS. Corticobulbar tract degeneration is known to occur with PBP, resulting in UMN signs and symptoms, such as jaw jerk reflex, hyperactive gag response, spasticity, and disinhibition of complex motor behaviors (e.g., laughter and crying) (Caroscio et al., 1987). Asymmetry with observations of weakness and cranial nerve impairments are relatively common (Caroscio et al., 1987), and most likely are related to asymmetry with the disease progression and spread.

Despite the involvement of lower cranial nerve neurons, extraocular musculature innervated by cranial nerves III, IV, and VI usually are spared until late in the course of the disease (Rocha et al., 2005). In addition, although signs and symptoms associated with ALS and PBP predominantly are efferent in nature, there is evidence for some afferent involvement as well. For instance, reduced sensation to heat has been reported. Researchers, however, have not observed progression of sensory deficits, as has been observed with motor impairments (Theys, Peeters, & Robberecht, 1999). Although sensory

involvement in ALS has frequently been reported to be clinically insignificant relative to dysphagia associated with bulbar dysfunction, it may have clinical importance. For instance, reduced laryngeal sensation has been reported in more than 50% of persons with ALS (Amin, Harris, Cassel, Grimes, & Heiman-Patterson, 2006). In addition, other researchers report observations of silent aspiration in this population (Briani et al., 1998; Wright & Jordan, 1997), which most likely is indicative of reduced laryngeal sensation.

AMYOTROPHIC LATERAL SCLEROSIS

Signs and Diagnostic Criteria

Diagnosis of ALS is based on guidelines developed by the World Federation of Neurology (WFN) Research Group on Motor Neuron Diseases (Table 11–2). The diagnostic process for ALS is complex in that it requires confirmation of characteristic clinical findings, in conjunction with other laboratory tests to rule out disorders that can mimic ALS. ALS-mimic syndromes include postpoliomyelitis syndrome, multifocal neuropathy, endocrinopathies, lead intoxication, and paraneoplastic syndromes (Brooks, Miller, Swash, & Munsat, 2000). Based on the revised El Escorial diagnostic criteria for ALS, the diagnosis can fall into one of the following categories: clinically definite, clinically probable, clinically probable-laboratory supported, and clinically possible ALS (Brooks et al., 2000) (Table 11–3).

Diagnostic signs and symptoms associated with PBP are essentially the same as those for ALS, except that they are limited to bulbar musculature. Cranial nerve

Table 11–2. Revised El Escorial Research Diagnostic Criteria for ALS

The diagnosis of ALS requires the presence of:

1. Evidence of lower motor neuron (LMN) degeneration by clinical, electrophysiologic or neuropathologic examination
2. Evidence of upper motor neuron (UMN) degeneration by clinical examination, and
3. Progressive spread of symptoms or signs within a region or to other regions, as determined by history or examination.

Together with the absence of:

1. Electrophysiologic or pathologic evidence of other disease processes that might explain the signs of LMN and/or UMN degeneration, and
2. Neuroimaging evidence of other disease processes that might explain the observed clinical and electrophysiologic signs.

Source: Brooks et al., 2000.

Table 11–3. ALS Diagnostic Categories

All categories assume that other possible diagnoses have been excluded.

Clinically definite ALS:	Clinical evidence of UMN and LMN signs in the bulbar region and at least two spinal regions, or UMN and LMN signs in three spinal regions.
Clinically definite familial ALS— Laboratory-supported:	Progressive UMN and LMN signs in at least a single region and family history of an ALS-associated gene mutation, e.g., superoxide dismutase-1 (SOD1) or hexoseaminidase A/B deficiency.
Clinically probable ALS:	Clinical evidence of UMN and LMN sign in at least two regions with some UMN signs rostral to LMN signs.
Clinically probable ALS— Laboratory-supported:	Clinical signs of UMN and LMN dysfunction in one region, or UMN signs in one region, and LMN signs defined by EMG criteria are present in at least two regions.
Clinically possible ALS:	Clinical signs of UMN and LMN dysfunction are found in one region, or UMN signs are found in two or more regions, or LMN signs are rostral to UMN signs.

Source: Brooks et al., 2000.

involvement associated with PBP is typically most apparent in the nerves exiting from the lower portion of the brainstem, (Caroscio et al., 1987), that is, cranial nerves V, VII, IX, X, XI, and XII (Yorkston, Miller, & Strand, 2004). Common impairments associated with UMN and LMN involvement are listed in Table 11-4.

Table 11–4. UMN and LMN Symptoms in PBP and ALS		
	UMN only	*LMN only*
General signs/ symptoms	• Hyperreflexia • Loss of dexterity • Muscle stiffness or spasticity • Positional clonus • Slowness of movement • Hypertonia • Pseudobulbar signs 　– Spasticity 　– Emotional lability 　– Release reflexes (e.g., suck, snout)	• Weakness • Hypotonia • Atrophy • Fasciculations • Diminished reflexes

Source: Francis et al., 1999; Yorkston et al., 2004.

Communication and Related Issues

Because of the combination of UMN and LMN involvement, dysarthria associated with ALS and PBP is mixed with features of both spasticity and flaccidity. Specific characteristics will vary depending on the current severity, stage of disease progression, relative degrees of UMN versus LMN, and specific muscle involvement, and respiratory capacity and control. Initially, the person may present with mild speech changes that do not affect intelligibility. Early signs of bulbar involvement associated with ALS have been reported to include altered voice quality, slower speaking rate, and lower ratings of overall communication effectiveness (Ball, Willis, Beukelman, & Pattee, 2001). Hypernasality due to velopharyngeal weakness and impaired strength and coordination of respiration for speech and swallowing are other common findings seen relatively early. Over time, dysarthria may become more apparent and slowly can progress to

the point of anarthria (total loss of motor speech). Slowness of speed, increased effort, and fatigue often are related to muscle spasticity affecting articulation. Changes in tongue strength, range of motion (ROM), size, and shape have been reported to be highly associated with changes in speech production in bulbar ALS (DePaul, Abbs, Caligiuri, Gracco, & Brooks, 1988; Dworkin, 1986).

Voice changes associated with bulbar ALS are characterized by strained, effortful quality with tremor and/or flutter (rapid oscillation tremor). Despite these changes, many persons with ALS are able to phonate until late into the course of their disease (Hillel & Miller, 1989). Hillel and Miller (1989) reported that approximately 30% of persons with bulbar ALS present with impaired vocal fold abduction and passive paradoxic movements of the vocal folds late in the course of the disease. A histochemical study has revealed atrophic fibers in laryngeal musculature of persons with ALS, with particularly severe neurogenic changes in the posterior cricoarytenoid muscle, the major vocal fold abductor (Murakami, Yagi, Mizuon, & Nomura, 1990). Chen and Garrett (2005) completed a retrospective study examining laryngeal signs and symptoms for persons with bulbar ALS who were seen at a local neurology and otolaryngology clinic over an approximately 2-year period. Of 44 patients, 48% complained of voice-related symptoms, and 11% specifically noted harsh, spastic, or strained vocal quality. Others reported a breathy voice quality. Thirteen had laryngeal endoscopy (videostroboscopy) performed and, in accordance with the differences in perceptual symptoms and complaints, variations in the patterns of dysfunction of laryngeal movement were observed: incomplete adduction (50%), vocal fold bowing (33%); hyperfunction (25%), and reduced abduction (25%) (Chen & Garrett, 2005). Laryngospasm also reportedly has occurred for some, following triggers such as cough, reflux, and odors (Forshew & Bromberg, 2003). Thus, it is most likely that voice symptoms occur due to a combination of impairments in intrinsic laryngeal muscles, particularly weakness of the abductors, and spasticity that prevents smooth, rapid adjustments in vocal fold movement. These combinations of pathologies lead to the symptoms that often include strained, strangled, even wet voice, with possible strider and a predisposition to laryngospasm.

Slowness of speaking rate has been reported to be a key factor associated with symptom progression in ALS, as it has been shown to precede a more rapid decline in intelligibility that occurs within the next 2 to 6 months (Ball, Beukelman, & Pattee, 2004). Reduced intelligibility and other speech symptoms have been shown to precede and correlate with

functional impairments in swallowing (Strand, Miller, Yorkston, & Hillel, 1996).

Emotional lability (pseudobulbar affect) is a frequent symptom that affects one's ability to control laughter and/or crying, a problem that interferes with speaking for some. It also is correlated with bulbar involvement (Newson-Davis, Abrahams, Goldstein, & Leigh, 1999). Pseudobulbar affect is believed to be a consequence of involvement of bilateral corticobulbar tracts in the subcortical white matter and brainstem that results in a loss of inhibitory control over emotional responses (Montgomery & Erickson, 1987).

Evolution

ALS is a relentless and rapidly progressive disease. Initial onset is frequently insidious, asymmetric, and in a focal region of the body. Over time the weakness progresses and spreads to adjacent regions of the body. The pattern of progression will depend, in part, on the initial location of weakness, for example, spinal versus bulbar onset. The median survival time ranges from 20 to 48 months, but some with ALS survive more than 10 years. Older age and bulbar onset are associated with poorer prognosis (Chio et al., 2009). The most common cause of death is respiratory failure.

Epidemiology

Incidence and prevalence of sporadic ALS has increased over the past several decades (Worms, 2001) perhaps due to improvements in diagnostic recognition and reporting. In the 1990s, average incidence of sporadic ALS was 1.89 per

100,000 per year, and the average prevalence was 5.2 per 100,000 (Worms, 2001). About two-thirds of ALS cases have a spinal onset, that is, classical "Charcot ALS" (Wijesekera & Leigh, 2009). Classical ALS tends to affect more males than females, with a male to female ratio of approximately 1.5 to 1 (Wijesekera & Leigh, 2009). The average age of sporadic ALS onset ranges between 55 to 65 years old (Haverkamp, Appel, & Appel, 1995; Wijesekera & Leigh, 2009). Approximately 5 to 10% of ALS cases are familial; of these, 20% are associated with a mutation of the SOD1 gene. In those with familial ALS, onset age tends to be about 10 years earlier than for those with sporadic ALS, and the male to female ratio is 1 to 1 (Wijesekera & Leigh, 2009).

Many persons diagnosed with ALS present with and maintain normal cognitive skills. However, approximately five percent of persons with ALS will have a concomitant frontotemporal dementia (FTD). For these persons, cognitive changes are evident and significantly affect evaluation, intervention, and outcomes. In a larger percentage of cases, however, there are more subtle impairments of executive functions that do not meet criteria for FTD (Lomen-Hoerth et al., 2003).

There are a few epidemiologic factors that distinguish bulbar onset ALS, aka PBP, from classic ALS. First, PBP has been reported to occur more frequently with increasing age (Forbes, Colville, & Swingler, 2004; Haverkamp et al.,1995). Forbes and associates (2004) reported that 50% of persons 80 years and older who were diagnosed with ALS presented with bulbar onset. Additionally, unlike classic ALS, PBP has been observed to occur more frequently with women than men (Caroscio et al., 1987; Haverkamp et al., 1995). In classic ALS, the male to female ratio is

3 to 2. However, PBP tends to affect older females more frequently, with a male to female ratio of 1 to 1 (Leigh et al., 2003). Cognitive/executive function impairments associated with frontal lobe involvement have been reported to be more pronounced for persons with pseudobulbar palsy symptoms (Abrahams et al., 1997; Schreiber et al., 2005). Finally, survival time for persons with PBP tends to be less than for ALS with spinal onset (Rocha et al., 2005).

Medical/Surgical Treatment

Presently, there is no cure for MNDs. Efforts of medical intervention are focused on slowing disease progression to increase length of survival, prophylactically minimizing the risk for secondary sequelae of MND, maintaining quality of life, and facilitating the person's ability to make informed choices throughout disease progression. The only medication currently FDA approved for treatment of ALS is the glutamate modulating agent, riluzole (Rilutek®). Clinical trials using this drug have shown marginal slowing of disease progression in some subjects (Leigh et al., 2003). Of utmost significance for persons with ALS is the management of respiration, nutrition and communication.

Swallowing in ALS and/or PBP

Epidemiology

Dysphagia is an ever present symptom for patients with bulbar involvement in ALS. However, dysphagia can also occur for those with predominantly spinal involvement ALS, due to impaired cough and respiratory symptoms. Increased severity of dysphagia is associated with increased bulbar symptoms as measured by the ALSFRS-R bulbar subscale (Fattori et al., 2006).

Pathology

The pathophysiology of dysphagia in ALS is characterized by weakness and incoordination of swallowing musculature, potentially affecting the oral, pharyngeal, and upper esophageal stages of swallowing. Disparities between the timing of voluntary movements and/or delayed initiation of automatic, patterned movements, with brisk and, at times, hyperreflexive actions, contribute to reduced coordination of the swallowing mechanism. ALS frequently progresses in a manner such that some muscle groups are more affected and slower moving than other muscle groups. Weakness and movement problems result from a combination of spasticity and flaccidity in the swallowing musculature. These seemingly opposite muscle tone conditions can affect even a single structure. For example, intrinsic muscles of the tongue may be significantly weakened by atrophying muscle fibers, whereas spasticity of extrinsic muscles contributes to overall slowing of lingual movements. In early stages of ALS, spasticity might be the predominant feature affecting range of motion and speed of movement. As the disease progresses, atrophy may predominate and overwhelm the involved muscles, in which case the presence of spasticity will no longer be a significant factor with regard to function.

Common oral stage difficulties include reduced speed of eating/swallowing, spontaneous reduction in sip and bite sizes, oral leakage, dry mouth, pocketing of food in the oral or buccal cavities, difficulty chewing, leakage from the mouth, reduced oral control of the bolus due to tongue weakness, and reduced transport efficiency. Common pharyngeal stage difficulties include incomplete laryngeal elevation and/or delayed initiation of the swallow (usually worse with volitional dry swallows), reduced glottic coordination with coughing and throat clearing, reduced management of secretions, and, more rarely, nasal regurgitation.

Reduced coordination of the various aspects and stages of the swallow often occur. Aspiration pneumonia typically is not an early symptom, likely due to the gradual progression of dysphagia (Yorkston et al., 2004). Coughing and choking are common in this group and are associated with degenerative changes in musculature used for speech, respiration, and swallowing; however, the presence of coughing and choking has not been correlated with pneumonia or chest infection for persons with MND (Hadjikoutis, Eccles, & Wiles, 2000). This finding may reflect the positive and protective aspects of coughing.

MNDs may also affect esophageal motility and upper esophageal sphincter (UES) dysfunction. For some, this can result in gastroesophageal reflux and/or a tendency for foods to "stick" or pool above the level of the UES. UES spasm occurs for some patients with ALS, but has not been correlated with disease progression (Higo, Tayama, Watanabe, & Nitou, 2002). Ertekin et al. (2000) described hypertonicity of the cricopharyngeal muscle, the principal muscle of the UES, as contributing to swallowing incoordination with voluntarily initiated swallows. These investigators also observed delayed initiation for voluntary swallows, in contrast to preservation of spontaneous swallows, until the advanced stages of disease progression.

Weight loss and malnutrition may result in reduced muscle strength and immunosuppression, which can profoundly affect survival (Heffernan et al., 2004; Worwood & Leigh, 1998). It may contribute to a cyclical exacerbation of respiratory weakness, fatigue, ventilatory drive, and ability to rebound from the same (Hadjikoutis & Wiles, 2001). Risk factors for malnutrition in MND include bulbar involvement and dysphagia, as well as other factors including depression, anxiety, and the loss of mobility and independence (Heffernan et al., 2004).

Respiratory difficulties are almost invariable for persons diagnosed with ALS, contributing significantly to risk for aspiration and pulmonary complications and ultimately leading to death (Benditt & Boitano, 2008; Heffernan et al., 2006). This is true whether the patient has bulbar involvement or only spinal symptoms. Despite having no direct effect on the lungs, respiratory impairments associated with MND can occur in any aspect of the mechanical respiratory system, including respiratory centers located in the medulla and weakness of the respiratory musculature for inspiration and forced expiration (Braun, 1987). Incoordination of swallowing with respiration may also occur (Hadjikoutis & Wiles, 2001; Nozaki et al., 2008). Some may experience subclinical signs/symptoms of hypoventilation, such as awakening frequently while sleeping, chronic headaches, and fatigue (Lechtzin, 2006).

Saliva management and secretion clearance difficulties are common in PBP as dysphagia progresses beyond the mild stages. These difficulties tend to occur in two forms: overly thickened secretions or mucus, and sialorrhea or excess thin saliva and drooling. Thickened secretions can occur due to dehydration, mouth breathing, and/or drying of pooled secretions. Sialorrhea occurs as a result of impaired ability of the oral muscles to seal the lips, transport saliva to the back of the mouth, and swallow; it is not a result of overproduction of saliva (Andersen et al., 2005). With saliva/secretion management issues, avoiding the extremes between excessive dryness and excess secretions is critical: both can be detrimental to swallowing and increase the risk for pulmonary complications.

Inability to cough and clear secretions is another significant risk factor for aspiration and respiratory failure. Reduced management of saliva and secretions increases the risk for aspiration, and contributes to airway obstruction that in turn adds to breathing difficulty, as well as difficulty using noninvasive ventilation (Hadjikoutis & Wiles, 2001). Cough weakness may occur for different reasons in PBP compared to those with limb involvement ALS. For persons with limb involvement only, cough strength would be affected most by weakness of inspiratory and expiratory respiratory musculature. Those with PBP, however, may have normally functioning inspiratory and expiratory musculature. Cough effectiveness in this group is more affected by the weakened bulbar muscles and vocal folds. This results in reduced coordination of the muscular responses with airflow, and an inability to buildup adequate subglottal pressure and maintain upper airway patency during cough attempts (Hadjikoutis & Wiles, 2001).

Clinical Assessment and Intervention

Knowledge of diagnosis, approximate onset date, and focal CNS location(s) of onset aids in tracking disease progression and determining prognosis. Symptom rating scales can be useful for tracking disease progression and symptoms, and anticipating intervention needs. The ALS Functional Rating Scale-Revised (ALSFRS-R) (Cedarbaum et al., 1999) is a brief instrument that aids in documenting current disease symptoms and progression. The ALSFRS-R originally is based on and includes all items from the ALS Severity Scale (ALSSS) (Yorkston, Strand, Miller, Hillel, & Smith, 1993). The ALSSS provided four rating scales in the following areas: speech, swallowing, lower extremity function, and upper extremity function. The ALSFRS-R has expanded on this by including additional items such as salivation, handwriting, cutting food and handling utensils, turning in bed and adjusting clothes, climbing stairs, and, more recently, scales for respiratory function. The full ALSFRS-R scale is composed of four subscales encompassing the following functional areas: bulbar, fine motor (upper extremity), gross motor (lower extremity), and respiratory (Appendix 11–A). The ALSFRS-R currently is the most widely accepted and used functional outcome scale in research and clinical practice (Shefner, 2008).

Pertinent observations in PBP include evaluation of the tongue for evidence of fasciculations and/or muscle wasting, tongue strength and range of motion, velopharyngeal function, voice quality and intensity, respiratory strength and coordination, control of cervical musculature, and the initiation, timing, and completeness of laryngeal elevation during a volitional/dry swallow. Fasciculations, wiggly, wormlike twitches under the surface of skin or mucosa, are indicative of LMN involvement. Atrophy, or shrinkage of muscle mass, also occurs due to LMN dysfunction. Tracking changes in tongue range of motion and strength over time aids intervention decision-making. York-

ston et al. (2004) suggested use of a 5-point scale to measure tongue strength and range of motion; this scale ranges from a Level 5, indicating normal tongue protrusion and strength/range of motion extending to the buccal cavities bilaterally, Llevel 1, indicating zero or minimal effective movement. Table 11–5 provides a list of frequently abnormal oral mechanism findings for persons with MND with associated potential clinical implications.

Examination of respiratory support should include observation for clinical signs/symptoms of hypoventilation, measures of vital capacity (VC) in upright and supine positions, and peak cough flow (PCF). Information about these measures can be found in Chapter 5. Measures of sustained phonation, spoken syllables per breath and perceptual voice quality provide information on respiratory support for speech combined with voice function.

Most of the common oral and pharyngeal phase dysphagia signs associated with PBP can be detected via the clinical swallowing examination (CSE). This may be insufficient if silent aspiration or significant UES dysfunction is suspected, however. Direct observations of eating and swallowing with various food and liquid types and viscosities must be considered within the context of the individual's overall risk for aspiration pneumonia (see Chapter 5).

Given the expense and potential discomfort associated with various means of instrumental evaluation, care should be given in determining necessity for, and type, of instrumental methods used to augment the CSE. A general rule in determining necessity is to consider whether the results will affect recommendations based on the clinical exam. For instance, if significant risk factors for aspiration are observed during the CSE, confirmation of such factors via an

Table 11–5. Frequently Abnormal and Clinically Significant Oral Mechanism Findings for Persons with MND

	Possible Abnormal Oral Mechanism Observations	Possible Clinical Swallowing Sequelae
Jaw muscles	• Temporal wasting • Reduced jaw excursion • Weakness of masseter and/or temporalis with bite	• Reduced ability to chew • Fatigue with chewing
Facial and labial muscles	• Weak facial muscles with smiling • Weak pucker • Reduced strength of lip seal • Evidence of fasciculations	• Oral leakage • Difficulty using a straw • Biting cheeks and/or tongue
Tongue	• Reduced ROM (range of motion): Protrusion and ability to reach to bilateral buccal cavities (cheeks) • Weakness with movements (may be different on each side) • Reduced speed • Evidence of fasciculations (wiggly, wormlike twitches under the surface of the mucosa) • Evidence of atrophy	• Reduced bolus control • Impaired oropharyngeal transit • Impaired initiation of pharyngeal phase swallow • Pocketing of foods in buccal cavities • Difficulty clearing pocketed foods from buccal cavities • Reduced control of thin liquids
Velopharyngeal muscles	• Weak or absent gag • Hyperreflexive gag • Weak or absent VP elevation with sustained phonation	• Gagging on solid foods (hyperreflexive gag) • Nasal leakage
Voice	• Reduced length of sustained phonation • Strained vocal quality • Tremor, flutter, and/or glottal fry • Reduced intensity	• Difficulty with glottic coordination with volitional and/or reflexive throat clear or cough to clear secretions • Laryngospasm • Partial glottic obstruction during cough and/or breathing efforts • Difficulty clearing secretions • Risk for aspiration
Volitional cough	• Reduced coordination • Weak/unproductive / Reduced Peak Cough Flow (PCF)	• Difficulty clearing secretions • Further risk for aspiration and pulmonary sequelae due to pooled secretions

Table 11–5. *continued*

	Possible Abnormal Oral Mechanism Observations	*Possible Clinical Swallowing Sequelae*
Vital capacity	• Reduced vital capacity (may be different in upright versus supine positions) (This can be difficult to measure with significant bulbar involvement due to poor lip seal, saliva management, and/or glottic obstruction.)	• If <50%, may have poor tolerance of surgical procedure for PEG placement
Oral cavity	• Oral dryness (xerostomia) • Poor oral hygiene	• Oral dryness and/or dried thick secretions can inhibit normal airway clearance of bacteria via the mucociliary escalator • Risk for aspiration pneumonia
Volitional dry swallow	• Delayed • Weak • Incomplete laryngeal elevation (may be more challenging with dry, volitional swallows)	• Difficulty clearing secretions • Risk for aspiration of secretions
Cervical muscles	• Neck extension at rest • Dropped head: Difficulty with holding the head upright	• Difficulty maintaining good position for swallowing • Difficulty with neck flexion posture

instrumental study likely will not alter recommendations or management of the problems. A related consideration in ALS, owing to anticipated progressive decline, is timing for instrumental evaluations. For instance, repeated use of a videofluoroscopic swallow examination (VFSE) to track disease progression would result in repeated exposure to radiation and ingestion of barium that potentially could have detrimental side effects. The most widely used instrumental methods of evaluating swallowing are the VFSE and endoscopic swallow examination. If significant UES tightness is suspected, manometry may be useful to evaluate pressure changes in the oropharynx, hypopharynx, and UES. To facilitate accuracy with differential diagnosis of dysphagia associated with ALS, information from all of the aforementioned components of the CSE and any indicated instrumental examinations must be considered and integrated into the assessment. Focusing on one or two components in isolation will increase the risk for diagnostic errors or clinically relevant omissions.

To date there is no treatment that has been shown to effectively improve swallowing impairments associated with ALS. However, behavioral and management strategies can be useful in prolonging comfort and safety with eating. Despite the ongoing progression of dysphagia, intervention is indicated for purposes of minimizing the risk for respiratory sequelae associated with swallowing, maintaining ability to eat/drink for as long as possible, secretion management, and, in conjunction with a nutritionist, advising the patient on the timing for a percutaneous endoscopic gastrostomy (PEG). In addition, strategies and counseling targeting maintenance of enjoyment and participation with social activities that involve eating may be included within an intervention plan to facilitate quality of life.

During earlier stages of disease progression, and depending on the specific signs/symptoms of dysphagia, a variety of strategies might be appropriate to aid the person's ability to eat safely as seen in Table 11-6. Swallowing maneuvers, such as the supraglottic swallow, effortful swallow, and Mendelsohn maneuver frequently are more difficult to perform for individuals with significant bulbar involvement due to muscle weakness and incoordination. However, some have reported maneuvers such as the supraglottic swallow to be appropriate when dysphagia symptoms are mild (Kuhnlein et al., 2008). Sensory techniques such as thermal-tactile stimulation can be helpful for initiating a swallow when directly applied, but have not been shown to generalize beyond the direct application (Rosenbek, Robbins, Fishback, & Levine,

1991; Sciortino, Liss, Case, Gerritsen, & Katz, 2003). In Table 11-7 we summarize recommendations for interventions in ALS and for each category indicate the level of evidence that is currently available. More detail regarding types of interventions that have been applied for specific impairments related to swallowing are provided in discussions below.

Exercise for Dysphagia Associated with ALS. The issue of whether or not to recommend exercise for persons with MND is controversial. Research findings in this area have been mixed. Generally, carefully monitored progressive resistance strengthening programs at submaximal levels of intensity and focused on muscles without significant weakness have been found to be helpful for some persons who have a slowly progressive disease course (Chen, Montes, & Mitsumoto, 2008; Francis et al., 1999). However, to date, no studies have demonstrated benefits of exercise for the oral or breathing musculature. Currently, literature examining the efficacy of exercises to strengthen oropharyngeal musculature in ALS is limited to two case studies (Dworkin & Hartman, 1979; Watts & Vanryckeghem, 2001). In both cases, the dysarthria worsened following the intervention. Watts and Vanryckeghem (2001) reported on the effects of speech and voice intervention for a female with bulbar ALS. Initially, the Lee Silverman Voice Treatment (LSVT) was applied with appropriate speech breathing patterns, and voice focus with resonant therapy. LSVT was reported to be ineffective; for this subject it resulted in reduced voice quality and ventricular phonation. Following LSVT, voice focus treatment and glottal fry techniques resulted in reduced ventricular compression less than 50% of the time.

Table 11–6. Behavioral Interventions for Dysphagia in ALS

Behavioral Intervention or Strategy	Concern or Observed Problems Addressed by the Strategy	Clinical Rationale
DIET MODIFICATION		
Food texture modifications (e.g., softer, cohesive foods)	• Difficulty chewing • Reduced oral control of bolus	• Soft cohesive foods are easier to chew and reduce risk for choking on stray chunks • Soft cohesive foods reduce risk for airway obstruction from large chunks of food.
Liquid viscosity modifications (e.g., nectar or honey thick liquids)	• Aspiration risk with thinner liquids (Caution: may increase risk for dehydration)	• Thicker viscosities move more slowly, therefore reducing aspiration risk for those with weakness and incoordination.
Medication intake modifications (e.g., break or crush meds in puree)	• Medications sticking in throat • Coughing with medications	• Reduces risk for choking and/or airway obstruction with swallowing pills
Avoid mixing food textures (e.g., soup with chunks of food)	• Reduced coordination and bolus control	• Reduces risk for aspiration of liquids or chunks.
Sensory enhancements	• Reduced sensation	• Cold temperature and/or carbonated liquids enhance sensation.
POSITIONING		
Upright position	• Aspiration risk with liquids or solids	• Facilitates proper position for swallowing and the effects of gravity on the movement of the bolus
Remain upright for a period of time after eating	• Signs/symptoms of reflux • Risk for aspirating pooled residue	• Minimizes or reduces reflux and/or tendency to aspirate pooled residue
Neck flexed (chin tilted slightly down toward chest)	• Maximize airway protection	• Mechanically aids in closing the airway.

continues

Table 11–6. *continued*

Behavioral Intervention or Strategy	Concern or Observed Problems Addressed by the Strategy	Clinical Rationale
Drinking through a straw	• Coughing associated with neck extension	• Facilitates maintaining a chin tuck position while swallowing liquids; minimizes need for neck extension (However, this requires coordination of sucking and swallowing.)
Drinking from a short cup or a nosey cup	• Coughing associated with neck extension • Inability to use a straw	• A shorter cup or a nosey cup minimizes the need for neck extension with drinking, and does not require a straw
Place food in optimal oral position for control	• Reduced tongue strength • Reduced bolus control	• Facilitates control of the bolus
Use of a soft collar (modified with for chin down positioning)	• Cervical weakness	• Maintain optimal positioning for swallowing and minimize fatigue.
AMOUNTS		
Small sips & bites	• Reduced swallowing speed and coordination	• Reduces aspiration risk.
One sip/bite at a time	• Reduced swallowing speed and coordination	• Reduced aspiration risk
OTHER STRATEGIES		
Double swallow	• Pooling in the valleculae or piriform sinuses	• Facilitates clearance of pooled residue in the valleculae and/or piriform sinuses
Slower speed (take your time)	• Incoordination	• Facilitates swallowing coordination
Energy conservation: Eat often (e.g., 6 smaller meals instead of 3), emphasize high calorie foods	• Fatigue	• Facilitates energy, safety, and strength with eating
Thorough oral care	• Poor oral hygiene • Tendency for oral residue	• Keeping the oral cavity clean reduces oral bacteria, and therefore risk for aspiration pneumonia

Table 11–7. Recommendations and Evidence for Swallowing Interventions in ALS

Type of Intervention*	Specific treatment(s)	Indications	Level of Evidence**
Strengthening exercises	Nonspecific oral-motor strengthening	Contraindicated	Expert opinion and case studies
Facilitation techniques	No data	Generally not recommended	Generally not recommended
Compensatory maneuvers and postures	Specific maneuvers and postures determined on basis of instrumental exams	Recommended	Expert opinion
Activity modification	Nonspecific diet modifications	Recommended	Expert opinion
Other	Cough retraining	Recommended	Expert opinion

*Defined in Chapter 7 (Principles of Intervention in Neuromuscular Disorders).
**Based on published reports.

Articulation treatment included oral motor motility and strengthening exercises. Intelligibility continued to decline despite the strengthening exercises. Intensive voice and articulation therapy was ineffective. Conversely, management techniques for dysphagia had a greater benefit in that it allowed for maintenance of oral intake and nutrition. Similarly, Dworkin and Hartman (1979) reported the case of a subject with bulbar ALS who showed no improvements following intensive intervention that included tongue strengthening exercises. Given the lack of supportive evidence, oral motor strengthening and other exercises such as the Shaker maneuver typically are not recommended for people with MNDs. These exercises may contribute to fatigue, and they have not been shown to halt or slow disease progression. Although emerging treatments such as electrical stimulation therapy have been promoted as appropriate for MND, currently, there are

no efficacy data and no clear physiologic reason to support its use in this population. As the MND progresses, energy conservation techniques are indicated.

Medical and Surgical Treatments for Dysphagia. Ideally, swallowing treatment occurs within the context of a multidisciplinary team, which may additionally include physicians from neurology, pulmonary, and otolaryngology, as well as professionals from respiratory therapy, nutrition, nursing, physical therapy, and occupational therapy. Interventions described below tend to occur collaboratively with such team members.

Laryngotracheal Separation Surgery. As bulbar involvement associated with ALS becomes more severe, chronic coughing on secretions can cause a great deal of discomfort. In order to alleviate these symptoms and eliminate aspiration, surgical interventions to separate the airway from the oropharynx are sometimes recommended. Total laryngectomy has been completed for some with severe bulbar involvement (Garvey, Boylan, Salassa, & Kennelly, 2009). An alternative to total laryngectomy is *tracheoesophageal anastomosis* (Figure 11-1) described by Lindeman (1975). This procedure involves a tracheal transection with the proximal end of the trachea diverted into the esophagus and the distal end brought to the skin to form a tracheotomy. Because this procedure is potentially reversible should the patient regain safe swallowing, it is considered by some a better alternative than total laryngectomy. For patients with progressive disease, however, this

typically is not an issue. Lindeman, Yarington, and Sutter (1976) modified the original procedure to eliminate the need to connect the trachea to the esophagus by closing the proximal trachea with a muscle flap. This *laryngotracheal separation* procedure (Figure 11-2) leaves a blind tracheal pouch where food and/or saliva potentially collects and pools. Suzuki et al. (2009) examined, via videofluoroscopy and subsequent lateral x-rays, the clearance of residue in the blind tracheal pouch in subjects with a variety of neurologic diagnoses that had undergone laryngotracheal separation surgery. For most subjects, the contrast residue in the tracheal pouch cleared within 24 hours,

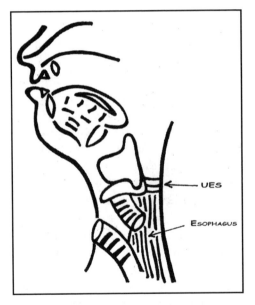

Figure 11–1. Lindeman's tracheoesophageal anastomosis. Tracheoesophageal anastomosis requires transection of the trachea with the proximal end joined to the esophagus and the distal end brought to the skin to form a tracheotomy for breathing. This potentially reversible procedure prevents pulmonary aspiration by diverting saliva or other material into the esophagus.

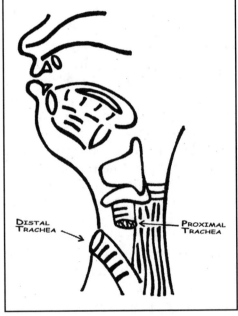

Figure 11–2. Laryngotracheal separation. To obviate the need to create an anastomosis of the trachea and esophagus, as is the case with tracheoesophageal anastomosis, the procedure was modified to create a blind pouch at the proximal end of the trachea.

although for others the contrast cleared between 48 to 96 hours later (Suzuki et al., 2009). No infections or other complications were observed. Conversely, other investigators have reported postsurgical complication rates that have exceed 40% (Zocratto, Savassi-Rocha, Paixao, & Salles, 2006). Despite some potential risk for complications, laryngotracheal separation in persons with severe bulbar ALS has been reported to be beneficial for quality of life, in that it reduces the fear of aspiration, the burden on caregivers and family members, and improves comfort and the ability to tolerate limited eating (Mita, 2007). It clearly has the potential to alleviate symptoms of constant coughing and choking on saliva, and maintains an airway for those experiencing airway obstructions due to laryngospasm.

A speech-language pathologist's pre- and postsurgical counseling and intervention is important to the education of patients on the benefits and caveats of laryngeal-tracheal separation procedures. These procedures result in a complete inability to phonate. For those with severe bulbar involvement, it is likely that intelligibility already will be severely impaired. Nevertheless, communication systems and strategies should ideally be in place before a separation procedure is performed. It also is important for patients, family members and caregivers to understand that this procedure does not guarantee return of swallowing. Although the procedure eliminates aspiration, it does not restore normal function to other components of swallowing, for example, tongue or palatal weakness. Some patients will be able to tolerate a modified diet following the procedure, but others will experience great difficulty with oral and pharyngeal transit and may experience sensations of gagging with anything other than small amounts of thin liquid. For those that experience gagging, coughing will no longer help, as the separated airway precludes this function. A videofluoroscopic swallow study following the procedure is needed to rule out leaks or fistula formation, and to determine the patient's ability to tolerate limited, recreational eating.

Secretion Management. Sialorrhea is often treated with oral or transdermal medications, such as amitriptyline (Elavil®), scopolamine (transdermal hyoscine), and/or glycopyrrolate (Robinul®) (Andersen, et al., 2005; Benditt & Boitano, 2008; Hillel & Miller, 1989). Side effects associated with medications should be monitored. Use of a home suction device is recommended to minimize risk of aspirating excess secretions. Botulinum toxin (BOTOX®) injections to the parotid glands, irradiation of the salivary glands, and surgical interventions have been utilized when medications and suctioning do not adequately address the problem; however, these are invasive interventions, each with the potential for complications (Andersen et al., 2005). For instance, there is some concern that botulinum toxin injections used for this purpose may further weaken already compromised musculature for speech, swallowing, and breathing (Leigh et al., 2003).

Treatment of thickened secretions must include efforts to maintain adequate hydration and minimize intake of caffeinated beverages. Maintaining adequate hydration and moist airway mucosa is also very important for functioning of the mucociliary escalator. Other helpful interventions might include use of a humidifier, avoiding foods known to cause thickened mucous and phlegm such as milk products, and use of medications that thin salivary flow (e.g., guaifenesin, an expectorant). The enzyme papase found in papaya and papaya juice has also been used to thin secretions.

Treatment for impaired cough effectiveness in ALS typically includes teaching the person and caregivers the Heimlich maneuver (for use in cases of emergency airway obstruction) and manually assisted cough techniques coupled with use of mechanical in-exsufflation (MIE). MIE has been reported to be superior to suctioning for clearing secretions, as it is noninvasive and therefore not traumatic to the soft tissues in the airway, and it can clear secretions distal to the large airways (Bach, 1993). MIE functions somewhat like a "shop-vac" for secretions. It delivers a large breath via facial mask or tracheostomy tube, followed by a strong, vacuum-like suction. When combined with manually assisted cough techniques, it can be quite effective. However, the effectiveness of this technique is frequently diminished in PBP owing to issues of glottic and airway obstruction previously described.

Treatment for UES Dysfunction.
Increases in UES pressure have been reported for some persons with MND. These findings have not been correlated with disease progression, but have been reported to be associated with increasing aspiration risk (Higo et al., 2002). Other studies have reported reduced coordination between the UES and muscles for laryngeal elevation characterized by delayed UES opening and a shorter duration of UES opening time (Ertekin et al., 2000). Myotomy and dilation procedures have been reported to be efficacious in treatment of structural disorders affecting UES, such as Zenker's diverticulum. However, they have not been proven effective for treatment of failed UES relaxation

occurring due to neurogenic dysphagia as the severity of UES dysfunction is heavily dependent on the function of the pharyngeal constrictor muscles (Cook, 2006). In addition, since dysphagia associated with ALS involves all stages of swallow function, rather than the UES in isolation, it often is not worth the risk of undergoing general anesthesia (Hillel & Miller, 1989).

Nutritional Management. Given the importance of adequate nutrition to survival and respiratory strength, interventions for dysphagia should be completed in conjunction with consultation from a nutritionist to facilitate evaluation and interventions related to maintaining nutritional status. The nutritionist can offer recommendations for adequate calorie intake and hydration within the constraints of the current diet modifications and swallowing precautions.

In 2009, the American Academy of Neurology published updated evidence based guidelines for the management of patients with ALS (Miller et al., 2009). The role of the PEG in the preservation of quality of life was emphasized. When a PEG is employed as a supplement for oral feedings, to maintain or increase energy, or to promote independence, it can have tremendous benefit. By anticipating the need and benefit derived from a PEG, clinicians can plan ahead and avoid having to make recommendations once the patient's condition has reached a crisis. In accordance with these guidelines, a PEG should be considered for the purposes of stabilizing weight and possibly prolonging survival. The guidelines also suggest that PEG be considered before forced vital capacity falls to below 50% of predicted to facilitate safety with patient tolerance of the procedure. As forced vital capacity continues to drop, the procedure becomes more risky.

Management of Velopharyngeal Insufficiency. A significant subset of individuals with ALS will experience velopharyngeal insufficiency. For these individuals, the speech pathologist should screen their candidacy for a palatal lift. Those who are good candidates tend to have a more flaccid (as opposed to spastic) palatal weakness, with a reduced gag response within the context of slower disease progression (Yorkston et al., 2001). In addition, they should demonstrate a difference in ability to produce plosives with and without nasal occlusion. In order to secure the palatal lift, adequate dentition typically is required. If the dysphagia and/or dysarthria is has progressed to the point of being moderate to severe, a palatal lift may not be beneficial.

SUMMARY

ALS is the most common form of MND. PBP is a form of bulbar onset ALS and a type of MND. Dysphagia is common in this population owing to the focal involvement of musculature innervated by lower cranial nerves. Even for those with limb onset ALS, dysphagia is a symptom for most. It is characterized by weakness and incoordination of the swallowing musculature. Dysphagia evaluation and intervention facilitates prolonged maintenance of overall health and quality of life.

REFERENCES

Abrahams, S., Goldstein, L. H., Al-Chalabi, A., Pickering, A., Morris, R. G., Passingham, R. E., . . . Leigh, P. N. (1997). Relation between cognitive dysfunction and pseudobulbar palsy in amyotrophic lateral sclerosis. *Journal of Neurology, Neurosurgery and Psychiatry, 62*, 464-472.

Amin, M. R., Harris, D., Cassel, S. G., Grimes, E., & Heiman-Patterson, T. (2006). Sensory testing in the assessment of laryngeal sensation in patients with amyotrophic lateral sclerosis. *Annals of Otolaryngology, Rhinology and Laryngology, 115*, 528-534.

Andersen, P. M., Borasio, G. D., Dengler, R., Hardiman, O., Kollewe, K., Leigh, P. N., . . . Tomik, B. (2005). EFNS task force on management of amyotrophic lateral sclerosis: Guidelines for diagnosing and clinical care of patients and relatives. *European Journal of Neurology, 12*, 921-938.

Bach, J. R. (1993). Mechanical insufflation-exsufflation: Comparison of peak expiratory flows with manually assisted and unassisted coughing techniques. *Chest, 104*, 1553-1562.

Ball, L. J., Beukelman, D. R., & Pattee, G. L. (2004). Communication effectiveness of individuals with amyotrophic lateral sclerosis. *Journal of Communication Disorders, 37*, 197-215.

Ball, L. J., Willis, A., Beukelman, D. R., & Pattee, G. L. (2001). A protocol for identification of early bulbar signs in amyotrophic lateral sclerosis. *Journal of the Neurological Sciences, 191*, 43-53.

Benditt, J. O., & Boitano, L. (2008). Respiratory treatment of amyotrophic lateral sclerosis. *Physical Medicine and Rehabilitation Clinics of North America, 19*, 559-572.

Braun, S. (1987). Respiratory system in amyotrophic lateral sclerosis. *Neurologic Clinics, 5*, 9-31.

Briani, C., Marcon, M., Ermani, M., Costantini, M., Bottin, R., Iurilli, V., . . . Angelini, C. (1998). Radiological evidence of subclinical dysphagia in motor neuron disease. *Journal of Neurology, 245*, 211-216.

Brooks, B. R., Miller, R. G., Swash, M., & Munsat, T. L. (2000). El Escorial revisited: Revised criteria for the diagnosis of amyotrophic lateral sclerosis. *Amyotrophic Lateral Sclerosis and Other Motor Neuron Disorders, 1*, 293-299.

Caroscio, J. T., Mulvihill, M. N., Sterling, R., & Abrams, B. (1987). Amyotrophic lateral sclerosis: Its natural history. *Neurologic Clinics, 5,* 1-8.

Cedarbaum, J. M., Stambler, N., Malta, E., Fuller, C., Hilt, D., Thurmond, B., & Nakanishi, A. (1999). The ALSFRS-R: A revised ALS functional rating scale that incorporates assessments of respiratory function. BDNF ALS Study Group (Phase III). *Journal of Neurological Science, 169,* 13-21.

Chen, A., & Garrett, C. G. (2005). Otolaryngologic presentations of amyotrophic lateral-sclerosis. *Otolaryngology-Head and Neck Surgery, 132,* 500-504.

Chen, A., Montes, J., & Mitsumoto, H. (2008). The role of exercise in amyotrophic lateral sclerosis. *Physical Medicine and Rehabilitation Clinics of North America, 19,* 545-557.

Chio, A., Logroscino, G., Hardiman, O., Swingler, R., Mitchell, D., Beghi, E., & Traynor, B. G. (2009). Prognostic factors in ALS: A critical review. *Amyotrophic Lateral Sclerosis, 10,* 310-323.

Cook, I. J. (2006). Clinical disorders of the upper esophageal sphincter. Goyal, R., & Shaker, R. (Eds.) *GI Motility Online* (10.1038/gimo037).

Czaplinski, A., Yen, A. A., Simpson, E. P., & Appel, S. H. (2006). Slower disease progression and prolonged survival in contemporary patients with amyotrophic lateral sclerosis: Is the natural history of amyotrophic lateral sclerosis changing? *Archives of Neurology, 63,* 1139-1143.

DePaul, R., Abbs, J. H., Caligiuri, M. P., Gracco, V. L., & Brooks, B. R. (1988). Hypoglossal, trigeminal, and facial motoneuron involvement in amyotrophic lateral sclerosis. *Neurology, 38,* 281-283.

Dworkin, J. P. (1986). Tongue strength measurement in patients with amyotrophic lateral sclerosis: Qualitative vs. quantitative procedures. *Archives of Physical Medicine and Rehabilitation, 61,* 422-424.

Dworkin, J. P., & Hartman, D. E. (1979). Progressive speech deterioration and dysphagia in amyotrophic lateral sclerosis: Case report. *Archives of Physical Medicine and Rehabilitation, 60,* 423-425.

Ertekin, C., Aydogdu, I., Yuceyar, N., Kiylioglu, N., Tarlaci, S., & Uludag, B. (2000). Pathophysiological mechanisms of oropharyngeal dysphagia in amyotrophic lateral sclerosis. *Brain, 123,* 125-140.

Fattori, B., Grosso, M., Bongioanni, P., Nacci, A., Cristofani, R., Alsharif, A., . . . Mariani, G. (2006). Assessment of swallowing by oropharyngoesophageal scintigraphy in patients with amyotrophic lateral sclerosis. *Dysphagia, 21,* 280-286.

Forbes, R. B., Colville, S., & Swingler, R. J. (2004). The epidemiology of amyotrophic lateral sclerosis (ALS/MND) in people aged 80 or over. *Age and Ageing, 33,* 131-134.

Forshew, D. A., & Bromberg, M. B. (2003). A survey of clinicians' practice in the symptomatic treatment of ALS. *Amyotrophic Lateral Sclerosis and Other Motor Neuron Disorders, 4,* 258-263.

Francis, K., Bach, J. R., & DeLisa, J. A. (1999). Evaluation and rehabilitation of patients with adult motor neuron disease. *Archives of Physical Medicine and Rehabilitation, 80,* 951-963.

Garvey, C. M., Boylan, K. B., Salassa, J. R., & Kennelly, K. D. (2009). Total laryngectomy in patients with advanced bulbar symptoms of amyotrophic lateral sclerosis. *Amyotrophic Lateral Sclerosis, 10,* 470-475.

Gautier, G., Verschueren, A., Monnier, A., Attarian, S., Salort-Campana, E., & Pouget, J. (2009). ALS with respiratory onset: Clinical features and effects of noninvasive ventilation on the prognosis. *Amyotrophic Lateral Sclerosis, 11,* 379-382.

Gordon, P. H., Cheng, B., Katz, I. B., Mitsumoto, H., & Rowland, L. P. (2009). Clinical features that distinguish PLS, upper motor neuron-dominant ALS, and typical ALS. *Neurology, 72,* 1948-1952.

Gordon, P. H., Cheng, B., Katz, I. B., Pinto, M., Hays, A. P., Mitsumoto, H., & Rowland, L. P. (2006). The natural history of primary lateral sclerosis. *Neurology, 66,* 647-653.

Hadjikoutis, S., Eccles, R., & Wiles, C. M. (2000). Coughing and choking in motor neuron disease. *Journal of Neurology, Neurosurgery and Psychiatry, 68,* 601-604.

Hadjikoutis, S., & Wiles, C. M. (2001). Respiratory complications related to bulbar dysfunction in motor neuron disease. *Acta Neurologica Scandinavica, 103*, 207–213.

Haverkamp, L. J., Appel, V., & Appel, S. H. (1995). Natural history of amyotrophic lateral sclerosis in a database population: Validation of a scoring system and a model for survival prediction. *Brain, 118*, 707–719.

Heffernan, C., Jenkinson, C., Holmes, T., Feder, G., Kupfer, R., Leigh, P. N., . . . Sidhu, P. (2004). Nutritional management in MND/ALS patients: an evidence based review. *Amyotrophic Lateral Sclerosis and Other Motor Neuron Disorders, 5*, 72–83.

Heffernan, C., Jenkinson, C., Holmes, T., Macleod, H., Kinnear, W., Oliver, D., . . . Ampong, M. A. (2006). Management of respiration in MND/ALS patients: An evidence-based review. *Amyotrophic Lateral Sclerosis, 7*, 5–15.

Higo, R., Tayama, N., Watanabe, T., & Nitou, T. (2002). Videomanofluorometric study in amyotrophic lateral sclerosis. *Laryngoscope, 112*, 911–917.

Hillel, A. D., & Miller, R. (1989). Bulbar amyotrophic lateral sclerosis: Patterns of progression and clinical management. *Head and Neck, 11*, 51–59.

Karam, C., Scelsa, S. N., & Macgowan, D. J. (2010). The clinical course of progressive bulbar palsy. *Amyotrophic Lateral Sclerosis, 11*, 364–368.

Kuhnlein, P., Gdynia, H. J., Sperfeld, A. D., Lindner-Pfleghar, B., Ludolph, A. C., Prosiegel, M., & Riecker, A. (2008). Diagnosis and treatment of bulbar symptoms in amyotrophic lateral sclerosis. *Nature Clinical Practice Neurology, 4*, 366–374.

Lechtzin, N. (2006). Respiratory effects of amyotrophic lateral sclerosis: Problems and solutions. *Respiratory Care, 51*, 871–881; discussion 881–874.

Leigh, P. N., Abrahams, S., Al-Chalabi, A., Ampong, M. A., Goldstein, L. H., Johnson, J., . . . Willey, E. (2003). The management of motor neurone disease. *Journal of Neurology, Neurosurgery and Psychiatry, 74*(Suppl. 4), iv32–iv47.

Lindeman, R. C. (1975). Diverting the paralyzed larynx: A reversible procedure for intractable aspiration. *Laryngoscope, 85*, 157–180.

Lindeman, R. C., Yarington, C. T., & Sutter, D. (1976). Clinical experience with the tracheoesophageal anastomosis for intractable aspiration. *Annals of Otology, Rhinology, and Laryngology, 85*, 609–613.

Lomen-Hoerth, C., Murphy, J., Langmore, S., Kramer, J. H., Olney, R. K., & Miller, B. (2003). Are amyotrophic lateral sclerosis patients cognitively normal? *Neurology, 60*, 1094–1097.

Miller, R. G., Jackson, C. E., Kasarskis, E. J., England, J. D., Forshew, D., Johnston, W., . . . Woolley, S. C. (2009). Practice parameter update: The care of the patient with amyotrophic lateral sclerosis: Drug, nutritional, and respiratory therapies (an evidence-based review): Report of the Quality Standards Subcommittee of the American Academy of Neurology. *Neurology, 73*, 1218–1226.

Mita, S. (2007). Laryngotracheal separation and tracheoesophageal diversion for intractable aspiration in ALS—usefulness and indication. *Brain and Nerve, 59*, 1149–1154.

Montgomery, G. K., & Erickson, L. M. (1987). Neuropsychological perspectives in amyotrophic lateral sclerosis. *Neurologic Clinics, 5*, 61–81.

Murakami, Y., Yagi, M., Mizuon, M., & Nomura, Y. (1990). A histochemical study of the intrinsic laryngeal muscles in amyotrophic lateral sclerosis (ALS). *Abstracts of the VIth World Congress of Bronchoesophagology, 5*(3), 171.

Newson-Davis, I. C., Abrahams, S., Goldstein, L. H., & Leigh, P. N. (1999). The emotional lability question: A new measure of emotional lability in amyotrophic lateral sclerosis. *Journal of the Neurological Sciences, 169*, 22–25.

Nozaki, S., Sugishita, S., Saito, T., Umaki, Y., Adachi, K., & Shinno, S. (2008). Prolonged apnea/hypopnea during water swallowing in patients with amyotrophic lateral sclerosis. Rinsho Shinkeigaku. *Clinical Neurology, 48*, 634–639.

Pascuzzi, R. M. (2002). ALS, motor neuron disease, and related disorders: A personal approach to diagnosis and management. *Seminars in Neurology, 22*, 75-87.

Rocha, J. A., Reis, C., Simoes, F., Fonseca, J., & Mendes Ribeiro, J. (2005). Diagnostic investigation and multidisciplinary management in motor neuron disease. *Journal of Neurology, 252*, 1435-1447.

Rosenbek, J. C., Robbins, J., Fishback, B., & Levine, R. L. (1991). Effects of thermal application on dysphagia after stroke. *Journal of Speech and Hearing Research, 34*, 1257-1268.

Schreiber, H., Gaigalat, T., Wiedemuth-Catrinescu, U., Graf, M., Uttner, I., Muche, R., & Ludolph, A. C.(2005). Cognitive function in bulbar- and spinal-onset amyotrophic lateral sclerosis. A longitudinal study in 52 patients. *Journal of Neurology, 252*, 772-781.

Sciortino, K., Liss, J. M., Case, J. L., Gerritsen, K. G., & Katz, R. C. (2003). Effects of mechanical, cold, gustatory, and combined stimulation to the human anterior faucial pillars. *Dysphagia, 18*, 16-26.

Shefner, J. M. (2008). Designing clinical trials in amyotrophic lateral sclerosis. *Physical Medicine and Rehabilitation Clinics of North America, 19*, 495-508.

Strand, E. A., Miller, R. M., Yorkston, K. M., & Hillel, A. D. (1996). Management of oral-pharyngeal dysphagia symptoms in amyotrophic lateral sclerosis. *Dysphagia, 11*, 129-139.

Strong, M., & Rosenfeld, J. (2003). Amyotrophic lateral sclerosis: A review of current concepts. *Amyotrophic Lateral Sclerosis and Other Motor Neuron Disorders, 4*, 136-143.

Suzuki, H., Hiraki, N., Murakami, C., Suzuki, S., Takada, A., Ohbuchi, T., . . . Shimono, M. (2009). Drainage of the tracheal blind pouch created by laryngotracheal separation. *European Archives of Oto-Rhino-Laryngology, 266*, 1279-1283.

Theys, P. A., Peeters, E., & Robberecht, W. (1999). Evolution of motor and sensory deficits in amyotrophic lateral sclerosis estimated by neurophysiological techniques. *Journal of Neurology, 246*, 438-442.

Watts, C. R., & Vanryckeghem, M. (2001). Laryngeal dysfunction in amyotrophic lateral sclerosis: A review and case report. *BioMed Central (BMC) Ear, Nose and Throat Disorders, 1*, 1.

Wijesekera, L. C., & Leigh, P. N. (2009). Amyotrophic lateral sclerosis. *Orphanet Journal of Rare Diseases, 4*, 3.

Worms, P. M. (2001). The epidemiology of motor neuron diseases: A review of recent studies. *Journal of the Neurological Sciences, 191*, 3-9.

Worwood, A. M., & Leigh, P. N. (1998). Indicators and prevalence of malnutrition in motor neurone disease. *European Neurology, 40*, 159-163.

Wright, R., & Jordan, C. (1997). Videofluoroscopic evaluation of dysphagia in motor neurone disease with modified barium swallow. *Palliative Medicine, 11*, 44-48.

Yorkston, K. M., Miller, B. M., & Strand, E. A. (2004). *Management of speech and swallowing in degenerative diseases* (2nd ed.). Austin, TX: Pro-Ed.

Yorkston, K. M., Spencer, K. A., Duffy, J. R., Beukelman, D. R., Golper, L. A., Miller, R. M., . . . Sullivan, M. (2001). Evidence-based practice guidelines for dysarthria: Management of velopharyngeal function. *Journal of Medical Speech-Language Pathology, 9*, 257-273.

Yorkston, K. M., Strand, E., Miller, R., Hillel, H., & Smith, K. (1993). Speech deterioration in amyotrophic lateral sclerosis: Implications for the timing of intervention. *Journal of Medical Speech-Language Pathology, 1*, 35-46.

Zocratto, O. B., Savassi-Rocha, P. R., Paixao, R. M., & Salles, J. M. (2006). Laryngotracheal separation surgery: Outcome in 60 patients. *Otolaryngology-Head and Neck Surgery, 135*, 571-575.

APPENDIX 11–A
The ALS Functional Rating Scale-Revised (ALSFRS-R)

BULBAR: ___/12

1. Speech

4 Normal speech processes

3 Detectable speech disturbance

2 Intelligible with repeating

1 Speech + nonvocal communication

0 Loss of useful speech

2. Salivation

4 Normal

3 Slight, definite excess in mouth (drool at night)

2 Moderate excess, minimal drooling

1 Marked excess, some drooling

0 Marked drooling, constant tissue/towel

3. Swallowing

4 Normal eating habits

3 Early eating problems, occasional choking

2 Diet consistency changes

1 Need supplemental tube feeding (+ oral)

0 NPO (no oral, exclusively tube-fed)

FINE MOTOR/UPPER EXTREMITY: ___/12

4. Handwriting

4 Normal

3 Slow or sloppy, all words are legible

2 Not all words are legible

1 Can grip pen, unable to write

0 Unable to grip pen

Complete only 5a or 5b, depending on feeding tube

5. a. Cutting Food & Handling Utensils (no tube)

4 Normal

3 Somewhat slow and clumsy, needs no help

2 Can cut most foods, some help needed

1 Food cut by someone else, feeds self slowly

0 Needs to be fed

b. Cutting Food & Handling Utensils (PEG)

4 Normal tube management

3 Clumsy, performs independently

2 Some help needed with closures & fasteners

1 Gives minimal assist to caregiver

0 Unable to perform any aspect of task

6. Dressing & Hygiene

4 Normal function

3 Independent, complete with ↑ effort

2 Intermittent assistance or substitute methods

1 Needs attendant for self-care

0 Total dependence

continues

Appendix 11–A continued

GROSS MOTOR/LOWER EXTREMITY: ___/12

7. Turning in Bed, Adjusting Clothes

4 Normal

3 Somewhat slow, clumsy: Independent

2 Can turn alone/adjust sheets, difficult

1 Can initiate, not turn/adjust sheets alone

0 Helpless

8. Walking

4 Normal

3 Early ambulation difficulties

2 Walks with assistance

1 Nonambulatory functional movement only

0 No purposeful leg movement

9. Climbing Stairs

4 Normal

3 Slow

2 Mild unsteadiness or fatigue

1 Needs assistance

0 Cannot do

RESPIRATORY: ___/12

10. Dyspnea (problems breathing)

4 None

3 Occurs when walking

2 Occurs when eating, bathing, or dressing

1 Occurs at rest, when either sitting or lying

0 Significant difficulties, considering mechanical respiratory support

11. Orthopnea (breathing problems laying flat)

4 None

3 Some difficulty sleeping at night due to shortness of breath, don't use >2 pillows

2 Need extra pillows to sleep (>2)

1 Can only sleep sitting up

0 Unable to sleep

12. Respiratory Insufficiency

4 None

3 Intermittent use of Bi-PAP

2 Continuous use of Bi-PAP at night

1 Continuous Bi-PAP day & night

0 Invasive mechanical ventilation by intubation or+ tracheostomy

TOTAL: ___/48

Source: Reproduced with permission from J. M. Cedarbaum, N. Stambler, E. Malta, C. Fuller, D. Hilt, B. Thurmond, and A. Nakashani. The ALSFRS-R: A revised ALS functional rating scale that incorporates assessments of respiratory function. BDNF ALS Study Group (Phase III). *Journal of Neurological Science,* 169, 13–21. Copyright ©1999 by the Society for Neuroscience.

12 Demyelinating Disease of the Central Nervous System (CNS)

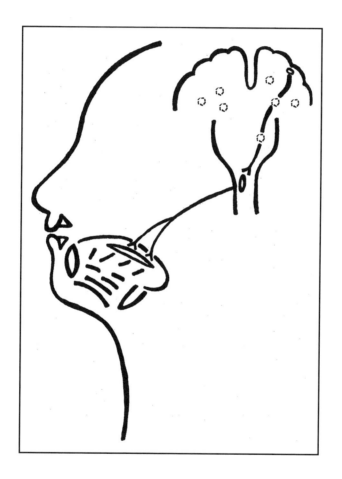

MYELIN

Myelin is a form of electrical insulation that covers the axons of neurons in the central nervous system (CNS) and peripheral nervous system (PNS). In appearance myelinated axons are white, and thus make up the white matter of the nervous system. Myelin is composed of about 80% lipid and 20% protein. Myelination of axons is the outgrowth from glia, the support cells of the nervous system. In the CNS, glial cells called oligodendrocytes form the myelin to insulate axons; in the PNS, myelin arises from Schwann cells.

As demonstrated in Figure 12–1, the myelin sheath is segmented with regularly occurring gaps approximately every two millimeters along the length of the axon called nodes of Ranvier. Functionally, these nodes serve to accelerate the speed of electrical impulses along the length of the axon. Rather than flowing continuously along the axon, as is the case in nonmyelinated axons, the segmented myelin allows for an action potential to jump from one node to the next. This process allows for a speed of propagation that is many times faster than that of a nonmyelinated axon. Furthermore, myelin acts like an insulation and helps to prevent the current from escaping the axon. In the presence of demyelinating disease, the affected axons degenerate and the associated neuron dies.

DEMYELINATING DISEASES

Demyelination refers to damage to or loss of this myelin sheath that protects the nerve fibers in the CNS or PNS. Loss or damage to myelin slows the speed of neuro-signal transmission along the axon, and eventually leads to axonal damage. Demyelinating diseases include those in which there is damage to the myelin sheath of neurons. Examples of diseases that result in demyelination of peripheral nerves include Guillain-Barré syndrome (described in Chapter 10, Peripheral Nerve Disease) and Charcot-Marie-Tooth disease. This chapter focuses specifically on demyelinating diseases of the CNS. Multiple sclerosis is the most common and well known of the demyelinating diseases of the CNS. Examples of other acquired diseases that result in demyelination within the CNS include neuromyelitis optica

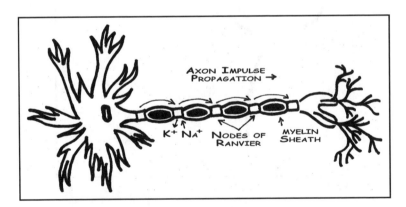

Figure 12–1. Neuron with myelinated axon. Segmented myelin coating supplied by oligodendrocytes in the CNS provide both for insulation to prevent a neural impulse from escaping the axon membrane and a means of faster neural impulse propagation. An impulse literally jumps from one node of Ranvier to the next, thus facilitating transmissions at velocities much greater than is found in unmyelinated fibers.

(also known as *Devic disease*), optic neuritis, transverse myelitis, and progressive multifocal leukoencephalopathy (PML). Several of these CNS demyelinating conditions may overlap. For instance, although optic neuritis and transverse myelitis are conditions that can occur in isolation, they also are frequently associated with a diagnosis of MS. Although the etiology for PML is distinct from MS, a small group of individuals with MS have also developed PML following administration of Natalizumab, a medication used to treat the MS (Berger & Houff, 2006). The bulk of this chapter focuses on MS, as this is the most common disease associated with demyelination in the CNS and the most common source of dysphagia in this group of disorders.

MULTIPLE SCLEROSIS

Definition

MS is an autoimmune neurodegenerative disorder that causes damage primarily to the *white matter*, or myelin, within the CNS, that is, within the brain and spinal cord. It is characterized by inflammation and chronic destruction of the myelin sheath. Long-term, MS eventually leads to permanent axonal damage and eventual neuronal death that contributes to irreversible neurologic impairment and disability (Dutta & Trapp, 2010; Trapp & Nave, 2008; Trapp et al., 1998). Although the exact cause of MS is unknown, it is well known that immune system dysfunction is involved (Cui, 2005; Trapp & Nave, 2008). Environmental factors and genetic predisposition are thought to contribute to the etiology as well.

Signs and Diagnostic Criteria

Several distinct types of MS have been delineated based on disease progression patterns (Table 12–1). Relapsing-remitting MS (RRMS) is the most common form of MS and is characterized by acute onset neurologic symptoms followed by periods of remission, that is, improved neurologic function. Most with RRMS eventually will experience a transition into a progressive form of MS called secondary-progressive MS (SPMS); although a small subset of approximately 15 to 20% will not. This small subset is said to have "benign" MS, that is, MS that remains mild indefinitely. Those with unrelenting, progressive symptoms from the onset have a primary-progressive MS (PPMS) form of the disease.

MS causes impairments in sensory, motor, autonomic, and cognitive functions. The types and severity of impairments vary greatly across individuals, in part depending on the location and severity of lesions within the CNS.

Sensory Symptoms

A variety of sensory symptoms may occur with MS (Rae-Grant, Eckert, Bartz, & Reed, 1999). Paresthesias, for example, tingling or numbness, and dysesthesias, for example, burning sensations, are common. Lhermitte sign and Uhthoff phenomenon are particularly common in individuals with MS (Compston & Coles, 2008). Lhermitte sign refers to an electrical sensation running down the back and limbs following neck flexion or extension and is reported by many with patients with MS. Uhthoff phenomenon refers to a transient worsening of neurologic signs and symptoms associated with heat. For example, on a hot day,

Table 12–1. Types of Multiple Sclerosis (MS)

Type	Progression Pattern	Approximate Percentages of MS Population
Relapsing-remitting MS (RRMS)	Intermittent exacerbations with relative neurologic stability between exacerbations	80–85%
Secondary-progressive MS (SPMS)	Slow progressive decline in function with fewer exacerbations, following a period (approx. 8–20 years) of RRMS	80% of RRMS
Primary-progressive MS (PPMS)	Progressive decline from the onset of MS, without exacerbations or remissions	15%
Progressive-relapsing MS (PRMS)	Slow progression from the onset, along with relapses	Rare
"Benign" MS	Very little progression following the initial attack (EDSS ≤3 after 25 years)	15–20% of RRMS

Sources: Brown, Severson, and Kraft, 2006; Ebers, 2006; Trapp and Nave, 2008.

after exercising, or following a hot bath, patients experience an exacerbation of symptoms or new signs appear. Other commonly reported sensory symptoms include pain, fatigue, and heat sensitivity (Crayton & Rossman, 2006).

Fatigue and Pain

The precise cause of fatigue associated with MS is not known. However, other co-occurring symptoms associated with MS may contribute to fatigue. Specifically, selective muscle weakness, depression of mood, the impact of heat on nerve conduction, and the fact that more energy is needed for neural impulses to propagate along demyelinated fibers are all factors leading to the experience of fatigue. Medication side effects are also potential contributors to fatigue (Crayton & Rossman, 2006). Table 12-2 provides a selected list of medications frequently prescribed

for individuals with MS and describes their potential side effects.

Pain can be associated with disease related factors such as neuralgia, spasms, inflammation, and joint stiffness. Trigeminal neuralgia occurs for a small number of individuals with MS, and is said to be caused by demyelination at the nerve root entry zone or in the pontine trigeminal pathway in the CNS (Crayton & Rossman, 2006). Symptoms associated with MS tend to overlap and interact. For instance, spasticity may be the source of pain or exacerbate pain caused by other factors. In turn, medications used to control spasticity may exacerbate cognitive dysfunction and contribute to muscle weakness and fatigue.

Motor Impairments

Motor dysfunction may occur due to demyelination of axons from the upper

Table 12–2. Selected Medications Used to Treat MS Symptoms with Side Effects That May Exacerbate Dysphagia*

Medication	Common uses for MS:	Some common side effects that can affect swallowing safety
Baclofen: an agonist for GABA$_B$ receptors	Reduce spasticity	Drowsiness, fatigue, nausea, weakness.
Diazepam (Valium): a benzodiazepine derivative	Reduce pasticity, anxiety	Drowsiness, incoordination, fatigue, weakness, respiratory depression, cognitive changes
Clonazepam (Klonopin): a benzodiazepine anticonvulsant and muscle relaxant	Reduce spasticity	Drowsiness, incoordination, fatigue, increased saliva, cognitive changes
Tizanidine (Zanaflex), a centrally acting α-2 adrenergic agonist	Reduce spasticity	Drowsiness, weakness, numbness, incoordination, vomiting, dry mouth, heartburn
Gabapentin (Neurontin), an anticonvulsant	Reduce spasticity, seizures, neuropathic pain, paroxysmal symptoms	Drowsiness, weakness, shaking, cognitive changes, heartburn, dry mouth
Modafinil, an analeptic (i.e., CNS stimulant)	Reduce fatigue	Drowsiness, nausea, heartburn, loss of appetite, unusual tastes, dry mouth, excessive thirst, confusion, headache
Bupropion (Wellbutrin; Zyban), an antidepressant	Reduce fatigue	Drowsiness, dry mouth, nausea, vomiting, weight loss, shaking, headache
Caffeine (Ergotamine), a CNS psychoactive stimulant	Reduce fatigue	Stomach irritation, nausea, vomiting, bladder irritant (in context of MS)
Interferon	Reduce number of relapses	Flu-like symptoms (e.g., fever, chills, headache, nausea, diarrhea, vomiting, abdominal pain, joint aches, back pain, dizziness), tissue damage at the site of injection, depression, and fatigue
Ginko biloba	Improve cognition and reduce fatigue	GI discomfort, nausea, vomiting, headaches
Amitriptyline (Elavil), a tricyclic antidepressant	Reduce/manage depression	Drowsiness, dry mouth, confusion, headache, nausea, vomiting, weakness

*Selected medications are examples only.

motor neuron system (corticospinal and/ or corticobulbar tracts) and/or cerebellar system pathways (e.g., spinocerebellar, corticopontine-cerebellar, or vestibulospinal). Motor symptoms associated with MS include muscle spasticity, weakness, ataxia, tremor, dysmetria, and/or paroxysmal dystonia. Dysmetria is a tendency to over- or undershoot movement related targets or to misjudge the scale of movements required to accomplish a goal with the extremities and/or the eyes. Paroxysmal dystonia is a form of dyskinesia and refers to a rapid onset of an involuntary dystonic posture or a movement that is triggered by an extraneous stimulus, such as a loud noise, or by a self-generated rapid movement or another sensation (Crayton & Rossman, 2006).

Visual Impairments

Visual function can be disrupted due to sensory and/or motor impairments of the eyes (Chen & Gordon, 2005). Inflammation of the optic nerve due to demyelination of the axons within the nerve, or optic neuritis, may cause partial or complete loss of vision. Optic neuritis can occur as an isolated symptom or together with ocular motor impairments that disrupt the conjugate movements of the eyes. There are many forms of ocular motor impairments that range from mild weakness of intraocular muscles to complete internuclearophthalmoplegia (INO), or loss of horizontal gaze. Even mild weakness in the muscles that control eye movement can lead to double vision. Involuntary movements such as nystagmus, the spontaneous, rapid to-and-fro oscillations that occur in the eyes, or saccadic intrusions, an unintended drift of the eyes away from a target, can prevent a patient from maintaining a focused gaze. Balance difficulties may occur due to the combination of motor and visual impairments.

Autonomic Impairments

Autonomic nervous system (ANS) dysfunction is common in MS. Problems associated with changes in the ANS include bowel and bladder dysfunction, sexual dysfunction, and abnormal sweating responses. Impairments in cardiovascular autonomic reflexes, such as necessary blood pressure and heart rate adjustments to changes in position, are common.

Communication and Related Issues

Dysarthria has been reported to occur in approximately 40 to 51% of persons with MS (Hartelius, Runmarker, & Andersen, 2000; Merson & Rolnick, 1998). The most prominent characteristics of dysarthria associated with MS are reduced loudness control, vocal harshness, and imprecise articulation (Darley, Brown, & Goldstein, 1972; Merson & Rolnick, 1998). Hartelius et al. (2000) also reported vocal harshness, glottal fry, a reduced loudness level, changes in stress patterns, and generally reduced respiratory support to be among the most common characteristics of dysarthria associated with MS. Reduced loudness control can be a symptom of reduced respiratory support. In addition, there have been reports of rare instances where dysarthria has occurred specifically related to a loss of control over voluntary respiration (Noda & Umezaki, 1982).

Cognitive impairments are common in the context of MS. Estimated prevalence of cognitive impairments in MS is approximately 45 to 65% (Rao, 1995). Cognitive impairments in persons with MS are commonly characterized by mild-to-moderate deficits with attention and concentration, processing speed, recent memory, word-finding, executive functions, higher level reasoning and problem-solving, and visual-perceptual processing (Pepping & Ehde, 2005; Rao, 1995). Language deficits, general intelligence and certain types of memory (short-term and implicit) are relatively spared (Patti, 2009; Rao, 1995).

Diagnosis and Assessment

There is no single test that can confirm a diagnosis of MS. Rather, MS is diagnosed based on a combination of clinical observations, patient-reported history, and supportive laboratory findings. Objective laboratory tests required for diagnosis of MS include specific observations from magnetic resonance imaging (MRI), analysis of cerebrospinal fluid (CSF), and analysis of visual evoked potentials (VEP). The International Panel for MS diagnosis published diagnostic criteria in 2001 (McDonald et al., 2001). These are commonly known as the McDonald Criteria, named after the first author. Revisions to the McDonald Criteria were published by the International Panel for MS in 2005 (Polman et al., 2005). These revisions fine tuned the McDonald Criteria in accordance with current research and simplified some of the diagnostic criteria. The Revised McDonald Criteria are outlined in Table 12–3.

MRI is key to diagnosis of MS. The McDonald Criteria and associated revisions specify requirements for diagnosis that demonstrate MRI evidence of "dissemination in space and time." Generally, this means that observation of CNS lesions and relapses should be observed in a pattern that is separated in time and in scattered locations throughout the

white matter of the CNS. Table 12–4 presents specific MRI criteria to indicate dissemination in space. MRI findings are also useful to rehabilitation clinicians to aid clinical hypotheses about potential functional impairments.

MRI pathology associated with MS may be focal or diffuse (Simon, 2005, 2006). Focal lesions on MRI can range from small indications of edema to large lesions indicating demyelination or axonal damage (Simon, 2005). Diffuse pathology is more difficult to detect on MRI, but may be viewed indirectly as volume loss atrophy or identified with use of more advanced MRI methods; some diffuse pathology may go undetected on MRI (Simon, 2005, 2006). More advanced imaging techniques, for example, magnetization transfer imaging, can detect abnormalities in the "normal-appearing" white and/or gray matter. However, these methods are not typically available for clinical use. MRI enhancing techniques that include use of contrast agents and weighting methods that help to differentiate tissue type, for example, T1 and T2 weighting, are utilized to identify and characterize lesions in brain tissue. Acute, inflammatory lesions can be visualized on MRI with use of gadolinium-chelate, a contrast agent, with T2-weighted imaging. Enhanced lesions that are visualized following administration of gadolinium-chelate contrast indicate a disrupted blood-brain barrier and significant inflammation. Once the lesion ages beyond approximately 2 to 8 weeks, it typically no longer will be visible via gadolinium enhancement. The number and size of gadolinium enhancing lesions is variable over time within individuals (Simon, 2005). Focal T2 hyperintense lesions observed on MRI as bright spots do not indicate the specific underlying pathology; for instance, they may

Table 12–3. Revised McDonald Criteria for the Diagnosis of MS

Clinical Presentation	Additional data needed to confirm MS diagnosis
Two or more attacks; objective clinical evidence of ≥2 lesions	None (however, any additional data must be consistent with MS)
Two or more attacks; objective clinical evidence of one lesion	Dissemination in space, demonstrated by MRI (see Table 12–4 for MRI criteria). *or* Two or more MRI-detected lesions consistent with MS plus positive CSF* *or* Await further clinical attack involving a different site
One attack; objective clinical evidence of ≥2 lesions	Dissemination in time,** demonstrated by MRI *or* Second clinical attack
One attack; objective clinical evidence of one lesion (monosymptomatic presentation; clinically isolated syndrome)	Dissemination in space, demonstrated by MRI (see Table 12-4 for MRI criteria). *or* Two or more MRI-detected lesions consistent with MS plus positive CSF* and dissemination in time,** demonstrated by MRI or second clinical attack
Insidious neurologic progression, suggestive of primary progressive MS	One year of disease progression Plus two of the following: • Positive brain MRI (9 T2 lesions or ≥4 T2 lesions with positive visual evoked potential (VEP)) • Positive spinal cord MRI (2 focal T2 lesions) • Positive CSF*

*Positive CSF is determined by oligoclonal IgG bands in CSF, or a raised IgG index.

**MRI dissemination in time is demonstrated by a Gd-enhancing lesion at least 3 months following onset of clinical attack, if not at the site corresponding to the initial event, *or* detection of a new T2 lesion at any time compared with a reference scan done at least 30 days after the onset of the initial clinical event (Polman et al., 2005).

Source: Polman et al., 2005.

reflect edema, demyelination and/or axonal loss. Many T2 lesions will shrink over time leaving a smaller residual lesion ("T2 footprint"), thus indicating resolving edema and/or remyelination (Simon, 2005). Chronic T2 lesions may expand with disease activity. As MS progresses, T2 lesions increase in size and volume. T1 hypointense lesions, like the T2 lesions, can be chronic or acute. Chronic T1

Table 12–4. MRI Criteria to Indicate Dissemination in Space for MS Diagnosis
1. One gadolinium-enhancing lesion or nine T2-hyperintense lesions (if there is no gadolinium-enhancing lesion)
2. At least one infratentorial lesion
3. At least one juxtacortical lesion
4. At least three periventricular lesions
NOTE: A spinal cord lesion can be considered equivalent to a brain infratentorial lesion: an enhancing spinal cord lesion is considered to be equivalent to an enhancing brain lesion, and individual spinal cord lesions can contribute together with individual brain lesions to reach the required number of T2 lesions.

Source: Polman et al., 2005.

hypointense lesions, aka, "black holes," reflect more severe injury with axonal damage (Simon, 2005, 2006).

MRI detection of focal lesions associated with MS are known to have characteristic distributions (Simon, 2006), that is, dissemination in space. Lesions can be identified anywhere in the white matter of the brain or spinal cord. The lesions also may extend up to or into the gray matter. These are designated as juxtacortical, adjacent to gray matter, or juxtacortical-cortical, extending into gray matter (Simon, 2005). In the context of MS, it is rare to find lesions located entirely within the gray matter. Common findings include lesions in the periventricular white matter, corpus callosum, corona radiata, internal capsule, visual pathways, and centrum semiovale (the mass of white matter comprising the interior of the cerebral hemispheres). Common infratentorial lesion locations include the pons and other brainstem regions, cerebellar peduncles, cerebellum, and regions near the fourth ventricle. Observation of

brain atrophy is also common in MS, and most likely reflects myelin and axonal loss. Spinal cord lesions typically are characterized by asymmetric distributions, at times consistent with a partial transverse myelitis (inflammation occurring transversely across the width of the spinal cord) (Simon, 2006).

Although, tracking T1 and T2 lesions aids monitoring of disease progression in MS, the number of lesions has been reported to have a poor relationship with disability and clinical symptoms (Simon, 2006). This, in part, may be an artifact of current measurement tools. For instance, the most commonly used functional outcome measure for MS, the Expanded Disability Status Scale (EDSS), does not necessarily reflect all potential early MS symptoms as it is weighted heavily to reflect changes in mobility. It also is possible that clinical changes may become apparent only after a critical level of injury occurs (Simon, 2006). Imaging does not necessarily distinguish between the types of MS, that is, RRMS versus SPMS versus

PPMS (Simon, 2006). However, in PPMS there is increased evidence of atrophy and abnormalities in both white and grey matter, along with evidence of diffuse axonal loss and cortical demyelination (Miller & Leary, 2007).

Evolution

MS is a chronic, progressive, degenerative condition. Initially, MS typically presents as a sudden episode of neurologic impairment; the initial impairment may be motor, sensory, visual, or cerebellar (Ebers, 2006). Despite what is generally known about the various types of MS and reported average prognostic statistics, determining prognosis for an individual is extremely difficult, as the clinical course

tends to be highly variable between individuals. However, consideration of research on the natural history and evolution of MS can provide a broad sense of trends that have been observed.

Measuring Disease Progression in MS

A variety of measurement tools have been used to evaluate disease progression associated with MS, including some of the MRI measures described above and the rate of relapses. However, the most commonly used functional outcome measure of disease progression in MS is the Expanded Disability Status Scale (EDSS) (Kurtzke, 1983) as described in Table 12–5. Because the EDSS is the most widely used disability rating scale for individuals with MS, it is

Table 12–5. Expanded Disability Status Scale (EDSS)—As Defined by Kurtzke

Score	Description
0.0	Normal neurologic examination Grade 0 in all functional systems (FS); cerebral grade 1 acceptable
1.0	No disability with minimal signs in one FS (grade 1, excluding cerebral grade 1)
1.5	No disability with minimal signs in more than one FS (>1 FS grade 1, excluding cerebral grade 1)
2.0	Minimal disability in one FS (one FS grade 2, others 0 or 1)
2.5	Minimal disability in two FSs (two FS grade 2, others 0 or 1)
3.0	Moderate disability in one FS (one FS grade 3, others 0 or 1) or mild disability in three or four FS (three or four FS grade 2, others 0 or 1), though fully ambulatory
3.5	Fully ambulatory but with moderate disability in one FS (one grade 3) and one or two FS grade 2; or two FS grade 3 or five FS grade 2 (others 0 or 1)
4.0	Fully ambulatory without aid, self-sufficient, up and about some 12 hours a day, despite relatively severe disability consisting of one FS grade 4 (others 0 or 1), or a combination of lesser grades exceeding limits of previous steps; able to walk without aid or rest some 500 meters

Table 12–5. *continued*

Score	Description
4.5	Fully ambulatory without aid, up and about much of the day, able to work a full day, may otherwise have some limitation of full activity or require minimal assistance; characterized by relatively severe disability usually consisting of one FS grade 4 (others 0 or 1) or combinations of lesser grades exceeding limits of previous steps; able to walk without aid or rest some 300 meters
5.0	Ambulatory without aid or rest for about 200 meters; disability severe enough to impair full daily activities (e.g., to work a full day without special provisions); Usual FS equivalents are one grade 5 alone (others 0 or 1); or combinations of lesser grades usually exceeding specifications for step 4.0
5.5	Ambulatory without aid for about 100 meters; disability severe enough to preclude full daily activities; usual FS equivalents are one grade 5 alone (others 0 or 1) or a combination of lesser grades usually exceeding those for step 4.0
6.0	Intermittent or unilateral constant assistance (cane, crutch, brace) required to walk about 100 meters with or without resting (usual FS equivalents are combinations with more than two FS grade 3+)
6.5	Constant bilateral assistance (canes, crutches, braces) required to walk about 20 meters without resting (usual FS equivalents are combinations with more than two FS grade 3+)
7.0	Unable to walk beyond approximately 5 meters even with aid, essentially restricted to wheelchair; wheels self in standard wheelchair and transfers alone; up and about in wheelchair some 12 hours a day (usual FS equivalents are combinations with more than one FS grade 4+; very rarely pyramidal grade 5 alone)
7.5	Unable to take more than a few steps; restricted to wheelchair; may need aid in transfer; wheels self but cannot carry on in standard wheelchair a full day; May require motorized wheelchair (FS equivalents are combinations with more than one FS grade 4+)
8.0	Essentially restricted to bed or chair or perambulated in wheelchair, but may be out of bed itself much of the day; retains many self-care functions; generally has effective use of arms (usual FS equivalents are combinations; generally grade 4+ in several systems)
8.5	Essentially restricted to bed much of the day; has some effective use of arm(s); retains some self-care functions (usual FS equivalents are combinations, generally 4+ in several systems)
9.0	Helpless bed patient; can communicate and eat (usual FS equivalents are combinations, mostly grade 4+)
9.5	Totally helpless bed patient; unable to communicate effectively or eat/swallow (usual FS equivalents are combinations, almost all grade 4+)
10.0	Death due to MS

Source: Gaspari, Saletti, Scandellari, and Stecchi, 2009; Kurtzke, 1983.

important that swallowing clinicians are able to interpret the scores. However, there are a number of caveats associated with use of this scale. The EDSS is a relatively complex scoring system, administered by trained examiners, that incorporates ordinal ratings on a variety of functional systems (outlined in Table 12–6) integrated with ordinal disability status ratings. Primary scoring emphasis is placed on the individual's ability to ambulate. The EDSS is not sensitive to the range of changes related to cognition or pseudobulbar symptoms that might occur before more significant mobility impairments. Similarly, the EDSS and/or functional system ratings have not been found to be related to the severity of dysphagia (Abraham & Yun, 2002), with the exception of those for patients with progressive forms of MS and EDSS scores less than 6.5 (Calcagno, Ruoppolo, Grasso, De Vincentiis, & Paolucci, 2002). Dysarthria and dysphagia are attributed to the functional system titled "brainstem functions" only. It is important to recognize that this technically is an inaccurate designation

as these conditions can also result from impairments in other functional systems identified by the EDSS rating system, for example, pyramidal and cerebellar functions. The brainstem functional scale ratings are focused primarily on ocular movements and are inadequate for clinically meaningful ratings pertaining to speech and swallowing until these impairments become severe. Lower EDSS scores measured across relatively shorter durations, that is, 2 to 3 years, may not be sufficiently sensitive to clinically meaningful changes in level of disability (Ebers, 2006). These caveats make the EDSS difficult to interpret and of limited value for clinical decision-making. Despite these limits, the EDSS has been the primary measurement tool used to track disease progression patterns over the past several decades.

Disease Progression in MS

Disease progression associated with MS is highly variable between individuals. However, most with the diagnosis of MS

Table 12–6. Functional Systems

Functional System	Abbreviation	QA:
Pyramidal	p	Voluntary movement
Cerebellar	cll	Coordination of movement or balance
Brainstem	bs	Sensation and movement of the face/neck, and/or ocular movements
Sensory	s	Referring to parts below the head
Bowel & Bladder	bb	Retention or incontinence
Visual	v	Impairment of vision in the worst eye
Cerebral or Mental	cb	Memory, concentration, mood
Other/Misc.	o	May include other factors (e.g., fatigue)

Source: Kurtzke, 1983.

ultimately will experience progressive disability (Hauser & Oksenberg, 2006). Approximately 80 to 85% of individuals with MS are diagnosed as having the RRMS form (Ebers, 2006). The relapse rate is variable between individuals, but typically occurs at a rate of 1 to 2 relapses per year (Trapp & Nave, 2008). Approximately 15% will be diagnosed with a progressive form of MS, that is, PPMS, from the onset (Miller & Leary, 2007). The majority of individuals initially diagnosed with the RRMS form will transition into the SPMS form within approximately two decades (Ebers, 2006; Trapp & Nave, 2008). Not all individuals diagnosed with RRMS progress on to more severe disability. Some are said to have benign MS. Definitions for benign MS vary, but typically refer to an individual with RRMS maintaining an EDSS score ≤2 or 3 after 10 to 20 years disease duration (Tremlett, Zhao, Rieckmann, & Hutchinson, 2010). However, benign MS is transitory for some; for example, it is possible to maintain a low EDSS score for >10 years and then go on to develop higher levels of disability after this time. Those with a particularly rapid transition to severe disability (that is, EDSS >6) are sometimes referred to as having malignant MS (Tremlett et al., 2010). Individuals with a parent, sibling or extended family member with MS are classified as having familial MS. Familial MS does not necessarily predict disease severity, but has been associated with shorter times to secondary or primary progression (Tremlett et al., 2010), and a younger age of onset (Koch et al., 2008; Koch et al., 2010).

For most individuals with MS, prognosis has been largely related to age—age of onset and age at the occurrence of a progressive phase (Vukusic & Confavreux, 2007). Increased age and male gender are associated with poorer outcomes

(Tremlett et al., 2010). However, younger age at onset has been associated with an earlier onset of more severe disability (Tremlett et al., 2010). Those with younger age of onset tend to reach higher levels of disability (as measured by the EDSS) at a younger age (Vukusic & Confavreux, 2007). For those with RRMS, relapses typically decrease in frequency over time (Tremlett et al., 2010). Complete or near-complete recovery from the first attack and fewer relapses in the first five years have been shown to be related to a better prognosis, in other words, a slower progression to more significant disability or progression (Tremlett et al., 2010). However, the number and type of relapses in the RRMS phase do not necessarily predict long-term disability or progression after a progressive phase has begun (Tremlett et al., 2010).

Epidemiology

MS has been said to be "the most common cause of neurologic disability in young adults in the western world" (Tremlett et al., 2010). Onset of MS typically occurs in young adults between the ages of 20 and 40, and only rarely begins before age 10 and after age 60 (Rejdak, Jackson, & Giovannoni, 2010). More than 2.5 million individuals in North America and Europe have been diagnosed with MS (Trapp & Nave, 2008). Incidence rates are higher in women than in men, that is, 3.6 and 2.0 cases per 100,000 person-years, respectively (Alonso & Hernan, 2008). The female-to-male ratio has risen in recent years to 2.3 to 1. However, individuals with progression from the onset, that is, PPMS, tend to be about 10 years older and have a higher proportion of men, with a 1 to 1 male to female ratio (Miller & Leary, 2007).

Scientists have identified genetic and environmental factors that increase the risk for MS. Genetic factors associated with an increased incidence of MS include female gender, western European ancestry, and having an immediate genetically related family member diagnosed with MS (Rejdak et al., 2010). Environmental factors associated with increased risk for MS include living in higher latitude regions and acquiring common childhood infections at later ages, particularly mumps, measles, rubella, and Epstein-Barr virus (Compston & Coles, 2008). However, systematic review of epidemiologic studies has revealed an attenuation in the latitude gradient in MS, as the incidence of MS has increased in lower latitudes (Alonso & Hernan, 2008). Other environmental factors that have been proposed as possibly increasing risk for MS include smoking, environmental toxins, low sunlight exposure, vitamin D deficiency, dietary factors, and various forms of pollution (Compston & Coles, 2008).

Average life expectancy for individuals with MS is approximately 10 years shorter than the general population (Ragonese, Aridon, Salemi, D'Amelio, & Savettieri, 2008; Tremlett et al., 2010). Determining cause of death in the MS population is tricky, as many with MS may not die of MS-related causes. Furthermore, studies that retrospectively examine death certificates only are most likely biased, as MS is frequently not recorded on death certificates (Hirst, Swingler, Compston, Ben-Shlomo, & Robertson, 2008). Some studies report that MS is the most common cause of death in the MS population, presumably based on wording recorded in death certificates. However, given the overall heterogeneity of symptoms and the potential for second-ary complications associated with MS, determining which aspects of MS have contributed to premature death in these groups is unclear. Many studies report that the most common cause of death in the MS population is respiratory disease or infection, followed by cardiovascular diseases and cancers (Hirst et al., 2008; Ragonese et al., 2008). Death due to respiratory disease is more common in MS than the general population, whereas death due to cancer in MS groups has not differed substantially from that seen in the general population (Ragonese et al., 2008).

Medical/Surgical Treatment

Current medical interventions focus on the use of a variety of medications to treat acute exacerbations, manage specific symptoms, and/or to reduce the number of relapses. None of the current interventions to date have demonstrated an effect on the long-term course, that is, transition to a progressive form of the disease (Crayton & Rossman, 2006; Hauser & Oksenberg, 2006), nor have they proven effective for PPMS (Miller & Leary, 2007). Currently, there are no surgical interventions to treat or alter the course of the disease. Treatment for MS is extraordinarily complex in that the disease symptoms are frequently interrelated such that some symptoms may lead to exacerbation of other symptoms (Crayton & Rossman, 2006). In addition, many treatments targeting specific signs or symptoms in MS potentially can exacerbate or increase other signs or symptoms associated with MS. For instance, many medications used to treat various conditions such as spasticity have a side effect of drowsiness; this in turn can exacerbate the symptom of fatigue. Table 12–2 provides a list of commonly prescribed medications and common side effects that may contribute to dysphagia.

Acute exacerbations are frequently treated with corticosteroids, to reduce inflammation and promote remission (Crayton & Rossman, 2006). Disease modifying medications, such as interferons (interferon beta-1a, e.g., Avonex or Rebif; or interferon beta 1-b, e.g., Betaseron), glatiramer acetate, and mitoxantrone have been shown to reduce the number of relapses experienced by individuals with RRMS (Crayton & Rossman, 2006). Unfortunately, these disease-modifying interventions have not been shown to have an effect on transition to progressive forms of MS or the time frames to reaching higher levels of disability. Generally, interferons are naturally occurring proteins that can modify the response of the immune system. The specific interferons used in the treatment of MS differ from those used for other conditions, such as chronic hepatitis (Ogbru, 2010). There are a number of side effects associated with use of interferons, however, many of which may diminish with prolonged use. Side effects may include flulike symptoms (e.g., fever, chills, headache, nausea, diarrhea, vomiting, abdominal pain, joint aches, back pain, and dizziness), tissue damage at the site of injection, depression, and fatigue (Ogbru, 2010).

In addition to efforts to reduce and recover from relapses, a multidisciplinary team approach is indicated in treatment of MS. The expertise of specialists from a number of disciplines is required in order to apply interventions that attempt to slow disease progression, assist patients in coping with symptoms, prevent secondary complications, and maintain participation with functional activities for as long as possible.

Swallowing in Multiple Sclerosis

Epidemiology

Prevalence reports of dysphagia due to MS have ranged from 33 to 55% of the general MS population (Abraham, Scheinberg, Smith, & LaRocca, 1997; Daly, Code, & Andersen, 1962; Hartelius & Svensson, 1994; Klugman & Ross, 2002; Thomas & Wiles, 1999). Studies that examine prevalence of dysphagia in MS based on self-report instruments may be low estimates, as many with signs of dysphagia are not aware of it (Thomas & Wiles, 1999). Those with dysphagia due to MS frequently indicate a reduction in quality of life due to swallowing problems (Klugman & Ross, 2002). Although less frequent in the early stages of RRMS, as the EDSS scores rise to higher levels, percentages of individuals with MS related dysphagia increase substantially (De Pauw, Dejaeger, D'Hooghe, & Carton, 2002; Hartelius & Svensson, 1994; Thomas & Wiles, 1999). However, swallowing abnormalities have also been measured in groups with mild-moderate MS and mild or no dysphagia symptoms or complaints (Poorjavad et al., 2010; Wiesner et al., 2002). For instance, Poorjavad et al. (2010) reported dysphagia prevalence as high as 31.7% in individuals with mild-moderate MS, that is, EDSS scores ranging between 2 and 3.

Pathology

Patterns of dysphagia associated with MS are variable between individuals and can affect any phase of swallowing. Dysphagia in individuals with MS has been associated with involvement in the brainstem, cerebral/pyramidal, and/or cerebellar systems (Abraham et al., 1997; Thomas &

Wiles, 1999). Sensory loss associated with MS can increase the risk for an impaired cough reflex and silent aspiration. Factors such as vital capacity, depression, and level of disability have also been associated with dysphagia in MS (Thomas & Wiles, 1999). Cerebellar functional system involvement, in particular, has been reported to be a significant contributing factor in dysphagia in individuals with mild-moderate MS (Poorjavad et al., 2010). Similarly, disruption to the timing and sequencing of events associated with the pharyngeal phase of swallowing has been identified in individuals with MS across a range of severity levels (Abraham & Yun, 2002). Increased severity of brainstem involvement has been reportedly associated with dysphagia in individuals with MS (Calcagno et al., 2002). In addition, brainstem involvement has been specifically associated with laryngeal vestibule penetration (Abraham & Yun, 2002). As the number of lesions and extent of involvement increases, the risk for dysphagia also increases. Dysphagia can occur for many with lower levels of disability as measured by the EDSS, and most commonly involves the pharyngeal phase of swallowing (Poorjavad et al., 2010). As the EDSS scores rise to the higher levels and as limb impairments increase, percentages of patients with dysphagia dramatically increase (De Pauw et al., 2002; Hartelius & Svensson, 1994; Thomas & Wiles, 1999).

Dysphagia related complaints may include altered eating habits, coughing and/or choking, a sensation of food sticking in the throat, poor secretion management, poor oral-pharyngeal transit, and difficulty initiating a swallow (Daly et al., 1962; De Pauw et al., 2002; Hartelius & Svensson, 1994; Kirshner, 1989). In addition, self-feeding ability may be impaired

due to upper extremity paresis, tremor, and/or dysmetria. Abnormal oral mechanism findings may include phonatory impairments, a positive jaw jerk reflex, tongue weakness, cervical neck weakness, and abnormal ability to cough (Thomas & Wiles, 1999). Long- and short-term phonatory instability is also common in individuals with MS (Hartelius, Buder, & Strand, 1997; Konstantopoulos, Vikelis, Seikel, & Mitsikostas, 2010) and may play a role in patients' ability to efficiently protect their airway. Swallowing abnormalities detected via manofluoroscopy in individuals with MS have included impairments with oral bolus formation, delayed triggering of the swallow reflex, residue in the piriform sinuses and/or valleculae, impaired epiglottic tilt, repeated swallowing, penetration, aspiration, weakness of the pharyngeal constrictor muscles, and deficient upper esophageal sphincter opening (De Pauw et al., 2002). On videofluoroscopic swallow exam, most, but not all, persons with more severe MS have shown penetration, aspiration, delayed laryngeal elevation and pharyngeal constriction, and residue in the piriform sinuses (Wiesner et al., 2002). In addition, reduced pharyngeal peristalsis and delayed triggering of the swallow reflex have been observed in individuals with MS (Logemann, 1983). Upper esophageal sphincter tightness and esophageal dysmotility has been observed in as many as 50% of individuals with MS as well (Daly et al., 1962).

In the context of MS, it is important to distinguish between permanent versus transitory dysphagia. Permanent dysphagia refers to those having chronic symptoms in contrast to those whose symptoms are a result of an acute relapse. Transient dysphagia refers to a dysphagia that occurs in the context of a relapse and later resolves.

Respiratory Impairments in MS

In MS respiratory impairments may occur for a variety of reasons, including respiratory muscle impairments, pseudobulbar impairments, abnormalities in ventilatory control, and obstructive or central sleep apnea (Carter & Noseworthy, 1994; Fleming & Pollak, 2005; Howard et al., 1992). These impairments can occur at any time in the course of the disease and may differ depending on the location and number of lesions in the CNS. Acute respiratory failure has been associated with acute relapse for some (Carter & Noseworthy, 1994). There have been rare reports of severe respiratory impairments resulting in death relatively early in the disease course (Howard et al., 1992). During later stages of MS progression, respiratory involvement often is associated with the overall diffuse bodily neuromuscular systems (Morales & Gay, 2002). Respiratory impairments have been observed in approximately 63% of those with progressive forms of MS (PPMS and SPMS), and in 84% of those with severe cerebellar impairments (Grasso, Lubich, Guidi, Rinnenburger, & Paolucci, 2000).

Clearly, pseudobulbar impairments can result in respiratory concerns due to the risk for aspiration of food or liquids into the airway. The generalized body weakness found in patients with pseudobulbar symptoms frequently is associated with restrictive respiratory impairments. However, research that examined respiratory function in persons with MS who were ambulatory, and who were without bulbar impairments or respiratory complaints, also revealed significant reductions in respiratory volume and pressure measures (Altintas, Demir, Ikitimur, & Yildirim, 2007; Mutluay, Gurses, & Salp, 2005; Smeltzer et al., 1992). With respect to the pattern of impairment, measures of pressure were reduced more than volume measures, particularly for maximal expiratory pressure. Persons with MS without respiratory complaints were also observed to have weaker volume measures (forced vital capacity) in supine, as opposed to upright, position.

The inability to cough and clear secretions is a significant risk factor for aspiration and respiratory failure. Volitional cough weakness has been reported in MS and associated with the EDSS disability level score (Aiello et al., 2008).

Generally, studies have demonstrated a lack of correlation between disease duration and presence or severity of respiratory impairments (Buyse et al., 1997; Mutluay et al., 2005). In addition, several studies comment on the fact that persons with MS rarely complain of difficulty breathing, shortness of breath or other respiratory symptoms, even in the presence of significant, measurable respiratory impairments (Buyse et al., 1997; Mutluay et al., 2005; Smeltzer, Utell, Rudick, & Herndon, 1988).

Clinical Assessment and Intervention

Clinical assessment should begin with medical records review and gathering information regarding the history of the patient's medical condition. Gathering information regarding the individual's specific type of MS, approximate dates of diagnosis and symptom onset, onset symptoms, current symptoms, EDSS and FS scores, and MRI findings can be very helpful for developing clinical hypotheses for purposes of tracking disease progression and prognosis. This, in turn, aids appropriate planning for assessment and treatment. EDSS ratings (if available) can provide the clinician with a gross overall sense of disability, especially as it pertains to mobility. However, as indicated above, the EDSS may not specifically reflect changes associated with cognition or pseudobulbar impairments, including dysphagia.

The interview to obtain information regarding current symptoms should include questions about existing problems associated with swallowing, respiratory symptoms such as shortness of breath or dyspnea, and weight loss. Bergamaschi et al. (2009) developed a short, 10-item questionnaire that is a useful screening tool to detect the presence of dysphagia in individuals with MS: The *Dy*sphagia in *Mu*ltiple *S*clerosis (DYMUS). Individuals who indicate positive findings on any item in the questionnaire are candidates for further assessment. Particular items in this measure can also help direct the assessment. For instance, some items pertain to difficulty with liquids and others to solids foods.

Review of MRI findings in the brain and spinal cord can help to direct clinical hypotheses regarding functional impairments and subsequent assessment. For example, an observation of lesions in the cerebellum would suggest that the individual might experience ataxia. Observations of lesions in brainstem white matter would suggest an increase the individual's risk for symptoms related to speech and swallowing.

During the oral mechanism assessment for individuals with MS, it is important to assess components of function known to be affected with MS. Pertinent observations, therefore, would include sensation, movement and coordination patterns, voice quality and intensity, respiratory strength and control, control and positioning of the head and neck, as well as the initiation, timing and completeness of laryngeal elevation during a volitional swallow.

Given the variability in dysphagia-related signs and symptoms associated with MS, intervention decisions will vary depending in large part on the findings of the clinical examination. Unfortunately, there is very little research literature examining intervention for dysphagia associated with MS. Extant research is briefly summarized below and Table 12–7 outlines recommendations and levels of evidence for interventions as they apply to this population.

Compensatory strategies, such as modifications to posture, diet textures, and methods of eating have been effective for most patients with mild or moderate dysphagia related to MS (Calcagno et al., 2002). As cognitive impairments may contribute to aspiration risk, minimizing distractions and maximizing attention while eating will be appropriate. Furthermore, any techniques used to manage MS symptoms generally may also benefit swallowing, for example, maintaining a cool environment and avoiding excessive heat exposure. Energy conservation techniques are appropriate to manage fatigue, for example, eating smaller meals throughout the day and taking rest breaks.

Exercise is beneficial for improving and/or maintaining fitness and function for individuals with MS (Dalgas et al., 2010). However, it generally is recommended that exercise be modest and not taken to the point of extreme pain or fatigue. Respiratory muscle training targeting inspiratory and expiratory musculature to strengthen breathing and cough ability has been beneficial for individuals with MS as well (Fry & Chiara, 2010). However, there is no published research to date regarding the benefit of oral motor strengthening exercises for individuals

Table 12–7. Recommendations and Evidence for Swallowing Interventions in MS

Type of Intervention*	Specific treatment(s)	Indications	Level of Evidence**
Strengthening exercises	Nonspecific oral-motor strengthening—no data	Generally not recommended	Expert opinion
	Inspiratory and expiratory respiratory muscle strength training	Recommended	AAN Grade III
Facilitation techniques	NMES	Insufficient evidence	AAN Grade IV Generally, professional consensus regarding NMES is mixed.
Compensatory maneuvers and postures	Specific maneuvers and postures determined on basis of instrumental exams	Recommended	Expert opinion—AAN Grade IV
Activity modification	Nonspecific diet modifications	Recommended	Expert opinion
Medical	Botox to UES	Consider if UES tightness is a factor	AAN Grade III
	Vagal nerve stimulation (VNS)	Insufficient evidence	AAN Grade IV

*Defined in Chapter 7 (Principles of Intervention in Neuromusular Diseases).

**Based on published reports.

with MS. Literature discussing benefits of exercise in the limb musculature cannot be directly generalized to predict benefit in the muscles for speech and swallowing due to differences in muscle size, use, and composition.

One pilot study has been completed to date examining the use of neuromuscular electrostimulation (NMES) to treat dysphagia associated with MS (Bogaardt et al., 2009). Although small improvements in swallowing following NMES were reported for ≤50% of the 17 participants, for example, reductions in aspiration and residue in the piriform sinuses with liquids, the study had a number of important limitations. For instance, they did not indicate type of MS, nor did they control for the possibility of transient dysphagia occurring due to relapses and remissions. In addition, there were no comparisons with alternative forms of treatment and no control group. Therefore, further examination of the utility of NMES is needed to determine the benefit for individuals with MS.

Other more invasive experimental treatments for swallowing have been explored. One such potential treatment is vagal nerve stimulation (VNS). VNS involves electrical stimulation of the left vagus nerve via a stimulator implanted in the neck. Historically, VNS has been known as a treatment for intractable epilepsy. Recently, VNS has been experimentally applied to treat cerebellar tremor and dysphagia associated with MS (Marrosu et al., 2007). VNS was reported to improve speed of swallowing liquids, as measured by the 50-mL water-swallowing speed test (Marrosu et al., 2007). However, the study failed to show differences with intake of solids and definitive measures of aspiration or penetration were not reported. Furthermore, the 50-mL water-swallowing speed tests used to measure swallowing function in this study has been validated only with patient self-reports, not with gold standard methods of detecting aspiration such as videofluoroscopic swallow studies or fiberoptic endoscopic swallow studies (Nathadwarawala, McGroary, & Wiles, 1994; Nathadwarawala, Nicklin, & Wiles, 1992).

Botulinum toxin to the UES has been reported to temporarily reduce penetration and/or aspiration in a small group of individuals with MS. These patients all presented with hyperactive upper esophageal sphincter (UES) muscles (Restivo et al., 2010).

Severe dysphagia can lead to complications, such as aspiration pneumonia and/or malnutrition. Both of these complications can be life threatening and contribute to disease progression in MS. Therefore, when dysphagia associated with MS begins to progress to a chronic stage with higher risk for aspiration and/or malnutrition, it is appropriate to consider placement of a percutaneous endoscopic gastrostomy (PEG). For those with progressive forms of MS, it is best practice to consider PEG placement

before the patient develops severe respiratory impairment, as this will allow for better tolerance of the procedure.

PROGRESSIVE MULTIFOCAL LEUKOENCEPHALOPATHY (PML)

PML is demyelinating disease of the CNS that occurs in the presence of severe autoimmune dysfunction. It is caused by the JC polyomavirus (JCV), a virus that is present in a large proportion of the population, but only causes PML in the presence of severe immune system dysfunction. It typically is diagnosed based on detection of JCV in the cerebrospinal fluid, in the context of clinical symptoms and MRI findings consistent with PML; although the gold standard for diagnosis is brain biopsy. PML was considered a rare disease until the HIV/AIDS pandemic in the 1980s, when up to 5% of the HIV population developed PML. More recently, owing to highly active antiretroviral therapy for HIV/AIDS, these numbers have dropped and more have recovered to remission. However, PML has surfaced in some individuals with RRMS following treatment with the medication Natalizumab (Berger & Houff, 2006).

PML is similar to MS in that it is a demyelinating disease that destroys the myelin covering axons of nerves in multifocal regions of the CNS. However, there are several important factors that distinguish PML from MS. Progression in PML is much more aggressive than in MS, such that many with this condition will not survive beyond 3 months without aggressive medical therapies. Symptoms may include seizures, hemiparesis, visual impairments, cognitive dysfunction, speech dysfunction, and loss of balance (Berger & Houff, 2006). Unlike MS, language processing impairments are common (Berger, Pall, Lanska, & Whiteman, 1998). PML may lead to dysphagia. At this point, however, little is known about the prevalence and characteristics of dysphagia associated with PML.

SUMMARY

MS is the most common form of demyelinating disease of the CNS and the most common etiology of neurologic disability in young adults in Western countries. Other forms of CNS demyelinating disease that may affect swallowing include PML and neuromyelitis optica. The signs and symptoms associated with MS are variable between individuals and may affect all aspects of the neurologic system, that is, motor, sensory, cerebellar, autonomic, and cognitive. Treatment for MS is complex, in that interventions targeting specific symptoms may exacerbate others. Dysphagia associated with MS occurs for both mild relapsing-remitting and more progressive forms of MS. Dysphagia intervention contributes to improved overall maintenance of health and quality of life.

REFERENCES

Abraham, S., Scheinberg, L. C., Smith, C. R., & LaRocca, N. G. (1997). Neurologic impairment and disability status in outpatients with multiple sclerosis reporting dysphagia symptomatology. *Journal of Neurological Rehabilitation, 11*, 7-13.

Abraham, S., & Yun, P. (2002). Laryngopharyngeal dysmotility in multiple sclerosis. *Dysphagia, 17*(1), 69-74.

Aiello, M., Rampello, A., Granella, F., Maestrelli, M., Tzani, P., Immovilli, P., . . . Chetta, A. (2008). Cough efficacy is related to the disability status in patients with multiple sclerosis. *Respiration, 76*(3), 311-316.

Alonso, A., & Hernan, M. A. (2008). Temporal trends in the incidence of multiple sclerosis: A systematic review. *Neurology, 71*(2), 129-135.

Altintas, A., Demir, T., Ikitimur, H. D., & Yildirim, N. (2007). Pulmonary function in multiple sclerosis without any respiratory complaints. *Clinical Neurology and Neurosurgery, 109*, 242-246.

Bergamaschi, R., Crivelli, P., Rezzani, C., Patti, F., Solaro, C., Rossi, P., . . . Cosi, V. (2008). The DYMUS questionnaire for the assessment of dysphagia in multiple sclerosis. *Journal of the Neurological Sciences, 269*(1-2), 49-53.

Bergamaschi, R., Rezzani, C., Minguzzi, S., Amato, M. P., Patti, F., Marrosu, M. G., . . . Solaro, C. (2009). Validation of the DYMUS questionnaire for the assessment of dysphagia in multiple sclerosis. *Functional Neurology, 24*(3), 159-162.

Berger, J. R., & Houff, S. (2006). Progressive multifocal leukoencephalopathy: Lessons from AIDS and natalizumab. *Neurological Research, 28*(3), 299-305.

Berger, J. R., Pall, L., Lanska, D., & Whiteman, M. (1998). Progressive multifocal leukoencephalopathy in patients with HIV infection. *Journal of Neurovirology, 4*(1), 59-68.

Bogaardt, H., van Dam, D., Wever, N. M., Bruggeman, C. E., Koops, J., & Fokkens, W. J. (2009). Use of neuromuscular electrostimulation in the treatment of dysphagia in patients with multiple sclerosis. *Annals of Otology, Rhinology and Laryngology, 118*(4), 241-246.

Brown, T. R., Severson, B., & Kraft, G. H. (2006). Optimizing Your Medical Management. In R. Fraser, G. H. Kraft, D. Edhe, &

K. Johnson (Eds.), *The MS workbook*. Oakland, CA: New Harbinger.

Buyse, B., Demedts, M., Meekers, J., Vandegaer, L., Rochette, F., & Kerkhofs, L. (1997). Respiratory dysfunction in multiple sclerosis: A prospective analysis of 60 patients. *European Respiratory Journal, 10*(1), 139–145.

Calcagno, P., Ruoppolo, G., Grasso, M. G., De Vincentiis, M., & Paolucci, S. (2002). Dysphagia in multiple sclerosis—prevalence and prognostic factors. *Acta Neurologica Scandinavica, 105*(1), 40–43.

Carter, J. L., & Noseworthy, J. H. (1994). Ventilatory dysfunction in multiple sclerosis. *Clinical Chest Medicine, 15*, 693–703.

Chen, L., & Gordon, L. K. (2005). Ocular manifestations of multiple sclerosis. *Current Opinion in Ophthalmology, 16*(5), 315–320.

Compston, A., & Coles, A. (2008). Multiple sclerosis. *Lancet, 372*(9648), 1502–1517.

Crayton, H. J., & Rossman, H. S. (2006). Managing the symptoms of multiple sclerosis: A multimodal approach. *Clinical Therapeutics, 28*(4), 445–460.

Cui, J. Y. (2005). Multiple sclerosis: An immunologic perspective. *Physical Medicine and Rehabilitation Clinics of North America, 16*(2), 351–358.

Dalgas, U., Stenager, E., Jakobsen, J., Petersen, T., Overgaard, K., & Ingemann-Hansen, T. (2010). Muscle fiber size increases following resistance training in multiple sclerosis. *Multiple Sclerosis, 16*(11), 1367–1376.

Daly, D. D., Code, C. F., & Andersen, H. A. (1962). Disturbances of swallowing and esophageal motility in patients with multiple sclerosis. *Neurology, 12*, 250–256.

Darley, F. L., Brown, J. R., & Goldstein, N. P. (1972). Dysarthria in multiple sclerosis. *Journal of Speech and Hearing Research, 15*, 229–245.

De Pauw, A., Dejaeger, E., D'Hooghe, B., & Carton, H. (2002). Dysphagia in multiple sclerosis. *Clinical Neurology and Neurosurgery, 104*(4), 345–351.

Dutta, R., & Trapp, B. D. (2010). Mechanisms of neuronal dysfunction and degeneration in multiple sclerosis. *Progress in Neurobiology, 93*(1).

Ebers, G. (2006). Disease evolution in multiple sclerosis. *Journal of Neurology, 253*(0), vi3–vi8.

Fleming, W. E., & Pollak, C. P. (2005). Sleep disorders in multiple sclerosis. *Seminars in Neurology, 25*(1), 64–68.

Fry, D., & Chiara, T. (2010). Pulmonary dysfunction, assessment and treatment in multiple sclerosis. *International Journal of MS Care, 12*, 97–104.

Gaspari, M., Saletti, D., Scandellari, C., & Stecchi, S. (2009). Refining an automatic EDSS scoring expert system for routine clinical use in multiple sclerosis. *IEEE Transitions Information Technology in Biomedicine, 13*(4), 501–511.

Grasso, M. G., Lubich, S., Guidi, L., Rinnenburger, D., & Paolucci, S. (2000). Cerebellar deficit and respiratory impairment: A strong association in multiple sclerosis? *Acta Neurologica Scandinavica, 101*(2), 98–103.

Hartelius, L., Buder, E. H., & Strand, E. A. (1997). Long-term phonatory instability in individuals with multiple sclerosis. *Journal of Speech, Language, and Hearing Research, 40*(5), 1056–1072.

Hartelius, L., Runmarker, B., & Andersen, O. (2000). Prevalence and characteristics of dysarthria in a multiple-sclerosis incidence cohort: Relation to neurological data. *Folia Phoniatrica Logopaedica, 52*(4), 160–177.

Hartelius, L., & Svensson, P. (1994). Speech and swallowing symptoms associated with Parkinson's disease and multiple sclerosis: A survey. *Folia Phoniatrica et Logopedica, 46*(1), 9–17.

Hauser, S. L., & Oksenberg, J. R. (2006). The neurobiology of multiple sclerosis: Genes, inflammation, and neurodegeneration. *Neuron, 52*(1), 61–76.

Hirst, C., Swingler, R., Compston, D. A., Ben-Shlomo, Y., & Robertson, N. P. (2008). Survival and cause of death in multiple sclerosis: A prospective population-based study. *Journal of Neurology, Neurosurgery and Psychiatry, 79*(9), 1016–1021.

Howard, R. S., Wiles, C. M., Hirsch, N. P., Loh, L., Spencer, G. T., & Newsom-Davis, J. (1992). Respiratory involvement in multiple sclerosis. *Brain, 115* (Pt. 2), 479–494.

Kirshner, H. S. (1989). Causes of neurogenic dysphagia. *Dysphagia, 3*(4), 184–188.

Klugman, T. M., & Ross, E. (2002). Perceptions of the impact of speech, language, swallowing, and hearing difficulties on quality of life of a group of South African persons with multiple sclerosis. *Folia Phoniatrica et Logopedica, 54*(4), 201–221.

Koch, M., Uyttenboogaart, M., Heerings, M., Heersema, D., Mostert, J., & De Keyser, J. (2008). Progression in familial and non-familial MS. *Multiple Sclerosis, 14*(3), 300–306.

Koch, M., Zhao, Y., Yee, I., Guimond, C., Kingwell, E., Rieckmann, P., . . . Tremlett, H. (2010). Disease onset in familial and sporadic primary progressive multiple sclerosis. *Multiple Sclerosis, 16*(6), 694–700.

Konstantopoulos, K., Vikelis, M., Seikel, J. A., & Mitsikostas, D. D. (2010). The existence of phonatory instability in multiple sclerosis: An acoustic and electroglottographic study. *Neurologic Science, 31*(3), 259–268.

Kurtzke, J. F. (1983). Rating neurologic impairment in multiple sclerosis: An expanded disability status scale (EDSS). *Neurology, 33*(11), 1444–1452.

Logemann, J. (1983). *Evaluation and treatment of swallowing disorders.* San Diego, CA: College-Hill Press.

Marrosu, F., Maleci, A., Cocco, E., Puligheddu, M., Barberini, L., & Marrosu, M. G. (2007). Vagal nerve stimulation improves cerebellar tremor and dysphagia in multiple sclerosis. *Multiple Sclerosis, 13*(9), 1200–1202.

McDonald, W. I., Compston, A., Edan, G., Goodkin, D., Hartung, H. P., Lublin, F. D., . . . Wolinsky, J. S. (2001). Recommended diagnostic criteria for multiple sclerosis: Guidelines from the International Panel on the Diagnosis of Multiple Sclerosis. *Annals of Neurology, 50*(1), 121–127.

Merson, R. M., & Rolnick, M. I. (1998). Speech-language pathology and dysphagia in multiple sclerosis. *Physical Medicine and Rehabilitation Clinics of North America, 9*(3), 631–641.

Miller, D. H., & Leary, S. M. (2007). Primary-progressive multiple sclerosis. *Lancet Neurology, 6*(10), 903–912.

Morales, I. J., & Gay, P. C. (2002). Respiratory complications of poliomyelitis and multiple sclerosis. *Seminars in Respiratory and Critical Care Medicine, 23*(3), 267–274.

Mutluay, F. K., Gurses, H. N., & Salp, S. (2005). Effects of multiple sclerosis on respiratory functions. *Clinical Rehabilitation, 19*(4), 426–432.

Nathadwarawala, K. M., McGroary, A., & Wiles, C. M. (1994). Swallowing in neurological outpatients: Use of a timed test. *Dysphagia, 9*(2), 120–129.

Nathadwarawala, K. M., Nicklin, J., & Wiles, C. M. (1992). A timed test of swallowing capacity for neurological patients. *Journal of Neurology, Neurosurgery and Psychiatry, 55*(9), 822–825.

Noda, S., & Umezaki, H. (1982). Dysarthria due to loss of voluntary respiration. *Archives in Neurology, 39*(2), 132.

Ogbru, O. (2010). Interferons. *Medications and Drugs.* Retrieved October 26, 2010, from http://www.medicinenet.com/interferon/article.htm

Patti, F. (2009). Cognitive impairment in multiple sclerosis. *Multiple Sclerosis, 15*(1), 2–8.

Pepping, M., & Ehde, D. M. (2005). Neuropsychological evaluation and treatment of multiple sclerosis: The importance of a neuro-rehabilitation focus. *Physical Medicine and Rehabilitation Clinics of North America, 16*(2), 411–436.

Polman, C. H., Reingold, S. C., Edan, G., Filippi, M., Hartung, H. P., Kappos, L., . . . Wolinsky, J. S. (2005). Diagnostic criteria for multiple sclerosis: 2005 revisions to the "McDonald Criteria." *Annals of Neurology, 58*(6), 840–846.

Poorjavad, M., Derakhshandeh, F., Etemadifar, M., Soleymani, B., Minagar, A., & Maghzi, A. H. (2010). Oropharyngeal dysphagia in multiple sclerosis. *Multiple Sclerosis, 16*(3), 362–365.

Rae-Grant, A. D., Eckert, N. J., Bartz, S., & Reed, J. F. (1999). Sensory symptoms of multiple sclerosis: A hidden reservoir of morbidity. *Multiple Sclerosis*, *5*(3), 179–183.

Ragonese, P., Aridon, P., Salemi, G., D'Amelio, M., & Savettieri, G. (2008). Mortality in multiple sclerosis: A review. *European Journal of Neurology*, *15*(2), 123–127.

Rao, S. M. (1995). Neuropsychology of multiple sclerosis. *Current Opinion in Neurology*, *8*(3), 216–220.

Rejdak, K., Jackson, S., & Giovannoni, G. (2010). Multiple sclerosis: A practical overview for clinicians. *British Medical Bulletin*, *95*, 79–104.

Restivo, D. A., Marchese-Ragona, R., Patti, F., Solaro, C., Maimone, D., Zappala, G., & Pavone, A. (2010). Botulinum toxin improves dysphagia associated with multiple sclerosis. *European Journal of Neurology*.

Simon, J. H. (2005). MRI in multiple sclerosis. *Physical Medicine and Rehabilitation Clinics of North America*, *16*(2), 383–409, viii.

Simon, J. H. (2006). Update on multiple sclerosis. *Radiologic Clinics of North America*, *44*(1), 79–100, viii.

Smeltzer, S. C., Skurnick, J. H., Troiano, R., Cook, S. D., Duran, W., & M.H., L. (1992). Respiratory function in multiple sclerosis. Utility of clinical assessment of respiratory muscle function. *Chest*, *101*, 479–484.

Smeltzer, S. C., Utell, M. J., Rudick, R. A., & Herndon, R. M. (1988). Pulmonary function and dysfunction in multiple sclerosis. *Archives in Neurology*, *45*, 1245–1249.

Thomas, F. J., & Wiles, C. M. (1999). Dysphagia and nutritional status in multiple sclerosis. *Journal of Neurology*, *246*(8), 677–682.

Trapp, B. D., & Nave, K. A. (2008). Multiple sclerosis: An immune or neurodegenerative disorder? *Annual Review of Neuroscience*, *31*, 247–269.

Trapp, B. D., Peterson, J., Ransohoff, R. M., Rudick, R., Mörk, S., & Bö, L. (1998). Axonal transection in the lesions of multiple sclerosis. *New England Journal of Medicine*, *338*(5), 278–285.

Tremlett, H., Zhao, Y., Rieckmann, P., & Hutchinson, M. (2010). New perspectives in the natural history of multiple sclerosis. *Neurology*, *74*(24), 2004–2015.

Vukusic, S., & Confavreux, C. (2007). Natural history of multiple sclerosis: Risk factors and prognostic indicators. *Current Opinion in Neurology*, *20*(3), 269–274.

Wiesner, W., Wetzel, S. G., Kappos, L., Hoshi, M. M., Witte, U., Radue, E. W., & Steinbrich, W. (2002). Swallowing abnormalities in multiple sclerosis: Correlation between videofluoroscopy and subjective symptoms. *European Radiology*, *12*(4), 789–792.

Index